Praise for
Let's Get Physical

"Fact-packed but bouncy . . . Most enjo
light on less hallowed figures, like Jud
lessly upbeat founder of Jazzercise, who
of women's days'; and Bonnie Prudden
descendant of Davy Crockett. . . . [Frie
exercise, but for the right reasons: not slimming down but mood management, community, spirituality in the corporal."
　　—*The New York Times*

"Friedman's engaging stories of the women who created and transformed the fitness industry illustrate an evolution built upon strong
female shoulders."
　　—*The Washington Post*

"[A] fascinating look at the world of modern exercise and some of the
main female players in it."
　　—*New York Post*

"Canny and informative."
　　—*The New Yorker*

"Fascinating . . . Persuasively encapsulates the relatively recent history
of women's fitness and the wide-reaching impact its trailblazers had.
Let's Get Physical is packed with stories of people who come to classes
because of how they want to look, but stay because of how those
classes make them feel: strong, supported, engaged, and empowered."
　　—*The Atlantic*

"Danielle Friedman's new book, *Let's Get Physical: How Women
Discovered Exercise and Reshaped the World*, is basically a perfect
book. . . . The book uncovers an important history that was sitting
right there in the open but had never been wrapped between covers
and contextualized with the fitful fight for women's rights."
　　—Alexis Madrigal, *Forum* (KQED)

"There are few areas of American culture as complicated—and as understudied—as women's exercise. Which is why I feel like I've been waiting for a book like *Let's Get Physical* for decades: something that takes the history and importance of fitness *seriously*, but is also incisive and curious and readable and *fun*."
—Anne Helen Petersen

"Friedman takes a jaunt through the history of women's fitness in her astute and entertaining debut. . . . This zippy history is bursting with energy."
—*Publishers Weekly*

"Fascinating stuff."
—*Booklist*

"A fascinating and complicated history, masterfully shared. *Let's Get Physical* made me grateful to the women of the past and hopeful about the future of fitness. My favorite read of the year!"
—Kelly McGonigal, author of *The Joy of Movement*

"Danielle Friedman's wildly engaging *Let's Get Physical* answered the questions I didn't even know I had about the origins of women's fitness (Jane Fonda sold *how* many copies of her *Workout*?!), and left me with a huge debt of gratitude to the trailblazing women who had the foresight to do things like sneak into the Boston Marathon and invent the sports bra so that we could swan into the gym without a second thought. A fascinating, meticulously researched read that left me with a much greater appreciation for the burn of barre class."
—Doree Shafrir, cohost of *Forever35*
    and author of *Thanks for Waiting: The Joy
    (& Weirdness) of Being a Late Bloomer*

"It's easy to critique the class, race, and gender stereotypes perpetuated by many fitness industry advertising campaigns, but Friedman reminds us how revolutionary it was, not so long ago, to encourage women to do strenuous physical exercise. An engaging account of the complicated, unconventional individuals who pioneered today's fitness culture for women."

—Stephanie Coontz, author of *A Strange Stirring: The Feminine Mystique and American Women at the Dawn of the 1960s*

"It is all too easy to look at the history of women's fitness as an unconnected timeline of fads and celebrities. In *Let's Get Physical*, Danielle Friedman weaves together the cultural history of a movement that is nothing less than the story of the modern American woman—and she does it with fascinating and fun storytelling that will appeal to anyone who has ever wondered why thighs need to be mastered or buns should be made of steel."

—Dan Koeppel, author of *Banana: The Fate of the Fruit That Changed the World* and *Every Minute Is a Day: A Doctor, an Emergency Room, and a City Under Siege*

"A delicious deep dive . . . Danielle Friedman tracks exercise culture into the twenty-first century, debunking myths and delighting readers with diamond-sharp prose, wry humor, and rigorous research."

—Sarah Everts, author of *The Joy of Sweat: The Strange Science of Perspiration*

"Don't read this book because it's 'good for you.' Read it because it's an eye-opening cultural history of the fitness pioneers who put the 'move' into the feminist movement. *Let's Get Physical* reminded me of why feeling strong feels so good."

—Brooke Hauser, author of *Enter Helen: The Invention of Helen Gurley Brown and the Rise of the Modern Single Woman*

"How did we get from the notion that exercise was unladylike, even dangerous for women, to the 1980s fitness craze and beyond that has totally transformed women's lives? In this lively book, Danielle Friedman uses fitness pioneers and icons, from Bonnie Prudden to Jane Fonda to Lilias Folan, to trace how regular exercise became central to millions of women's pursuit of vitality, confidence, and happiness. Full of fun and inspiring stories, *Let's Get Physical* reminds us that this is not just a history of sports bras or leg warmers, but also of how feminism itself enabled and drew from women finding empowerment in the strength of their own bodies."

—Susan J. Douglas, author of *In Our Prime:*
How Older Women are Reinventing the Road Ahead

"Friedman's study of modern fitness culture is as illuminating as it is enthralling. She reveals the wild characters, political agendas, and social movements that changed not only our exercise behaviors but our understanding of exercise itself. Behind every workout there is a story, and it's usually a *good* one."

—Kelsey Miller, author of *Big Girl:*
How I Gave Up Dieting and Got a Life

"With lively writing and compelling storytelling—tales of bamboo swords, spandex, and a sexy gerbil included—Danielle Friedman teases out the complicated relationship between exercise culture and feminism in this engaging exploration of modern fitness history. You'll want to hit the barre afterward."

—Haley Shapley, author of *Strong Like Her:*
A Celebration of Rule Breakers, History Makers,
and Unstoppable Athletes

"This must-read book is an informative and entertaining read for any woman who has thought about getting fit."

—Zibby Owens, host of the *Moms*
Don't Have Time to Read Books podcast

Let's Get Physical

How Women Discovered Exercise
and Reshaped the World

DANIELLE FRIEDMAN

G. P. PUTNAM'S SONS | NEW YORK

To Daniel and Sam, for putting a spring in my step
and moving me beyond words;

to Jackie and Juliet, for lifting me up;

and to my parents, Richard and Karen, for everything.

PUTNAM
— EST. 1838 —

G. P. Putnam's Sons
Publishers Since 1838
An imprint of Penguin Random House LLC
penguinrandomhouse.com

The Library of Congress has catalogued the G. P. Putnam's Sons
hardcover edition as follows:

Names: Friedman, Danielle, author.

Title: Let's get physical: how women discovered exercise and
reshaped the world / Danielle Friedman.
Other titles: Let us get physical
Description: New York: G.P. Putnam's Sons, [2022] |
Includes bibliographical references and index.
Identifiers: LCCN 2021046686 (print) | LCCN 2021046687 (ebook) |
ISBN 9780593188422 (Hardcover) | ISBN 9780593188439 (eBook)
Subjects: LCSH: Exercise for women—History. | Physical fitness. | Feminism.
Classification: LCC GV482 .F75 2022 (print) | LCC GV482 (ebook) |
DDC 613.7/1082—dc23/eng/20211108
LC record available at https://lccn.loc.gov/2021046686
LC ebook record available at https://lccn.loc.gov/2021046687

First G. P. Putnam's Sons hardcover edition / January 2022
First G. P. Putnam's Sons trade paperback edition / January 2023
G. P. Putnam's Sons trade paperback ISBN: 9780593188446

Printed in the United States of America
1st Printing

Book design by Elke Sigal

A movement is only composed of people moving.
To feel its warmth and motion around us
is the end as well as the means.

—Gloria Steinem, *Moving Beyond Words*

Exercise gives you endorphins.
Endorphins make you happy.
Happy people just don't shoot their husbands.

—Elle Woods, *Legally Blonde*

Contents

INTRODUCTION

Sweat

Five years ago I walked into a Pure Barre studio for the most predictable of reasons: I was getting married. In a few months I would be wearing a strapless lace gown in a hotel ballroom in my childhood hometown of Atlanta. For one night, I would be in a literal spotlight.

I was marrying a wonderful man, and I had spent my career as a journalist making the case that women should be valued for their inner selves and not their appearance. But weddings have a way of stirring up our most basic desires, and even feminists sometimes fantasize about greeting the world with a flat stomach and firm arms.

My local barre studio on Manhattan's Upper East Side promised, in loopy letters on a sidewalk chalkboard, to LTB—lift, tone, burn—my then thirty-five-year-old body into that of a ballerina. Sounded highly improbable and completely perfect.

I was drawn to the studio in the same way I'd been drawn to my high school's cheerleading squad: desperate to join, but doubtful, in some core teen girl way, that I belonged. Or that I wanted to belong. This time, though, going for it wouldn't mean attempting a sad split in front of the popular girls—or giving up Model UN. So I slipped into the boutique fitness uniform of moisture-wicking everything, handed over my credit card, and swallowed hard.

When the class began, a ponytailed instructor wearing a headset microphone ushered me and a dozen other women to a ballet barre, where we moved our thighs *up an inch, down an inch* until our muscles trembled. On cue, I squeezed my "seat" (barre-speak for butt) until it spasmed and planked until I thought I might pass out. When I looked around the room, every other woman was stone-faced in her Lululemon. *Would one of them catch me if I collapsed mid-squat?* For the last few minutes, we lay on our backs and thrust our pelvises to a stripped-down version of Rihanna's "Umbrella."

At the end, I didn't die of embarrassment or exhaustion. I felt fantastic.

So I went back, again and again. The workout made me strong in parts of my body I hadn't realized were weak. It allowed me, for the first time in my life, to carry grocery bags without stopping to rest after three minutes. I didn't look like a ballerina, but I felt like one—light on my feet, energized, connected with my body in a totally new way. I came to understand that the other women in class weren't unfriendly but intensely focused, in the one space where they had to focus only on themselves. I, too, developed a resting barre face.

A few months into my new Pure Barre routine, I became curious: Where did the barre workout, which had become a phenomenon (and multibillion-dollar industry) in this country, come from? One internet rabbit hole led to another, and I discovered an origin story far richer than I was expecting. What had once seemed like a familiar rite of passage suddenly took on the feeling of a mystery waiting to be uncovered.

The workout was created in 1959 by Lotte Berk, a free-love

revolutionary and former dancer who wanted to help women improve their sex lives. (This explained why many of the exercises in class felt comically erotic, from pelvic tucks to a move called "knee dancing.") Almost as radical at the time, Berk encouraged women to use exercise to strengthen their body—to create a "corset of muscle." Her London studio was one of the first-ever boutique fitness studios, and she attracted a celebrity clientele of actresses, writers, and on one occasion Barbra Streisand, who allegedly never removed her hat.

I wrote about this history in a feature for *New York* magazine's The Cut titled "The Secret Sexual History of the Barre Workout," and the story went viral. Few of the workout's devotees, including studio owners and instructors, knew about its roots. Some were scandalized, while others were delighted. For me, however, researching the piece opened my eyes to more than one workout's wild origins: It felt like unlocking a portal to a hidden feminist history.

While fitness culture today can feel sleek and sometimes sterile, the story of how women's exercise developed in the twentieth century until now, I discovered, is weird and messy and awkward and glamorous. It's rich with cinematic characters and forgotten pioneers of what we now call self-care. But more than that, it's the story of a paradigm shift in the way women, so long accepted as the "weaker sex," came to view their bodies. Because when women first began exercising en masse, they were participating in something subversive: the cultivation of physical strength and autonomy.

Today, I exercise for energy, for strength, and for my mental health. I exercise to feel the endorphin high of accomplishment and to manage life's lows. I exercise to remind myself I can persevere. And I am not alone. Most of the women I know—as well as the many women across the country I interviewed for this book—consider regular physical activity essential to their emotional and physical well-being.

My mom, who is in her early seventies, calls her weekly cardio dance classes a "surefire source of joy."

Before the coronavirus pandemic, some 73 million Americans belonged to at least one gym, studio, or health club. The pandemic shook the fitness industry, forcing nearly 20 percent of brick-and-mortar spaces to permanently close. But it also led to a dramatic rise in home exercise: By mid-2020, more than 80 percent of fitness consumers had livestreamed workouts, compared with only 7 percent before the global lockdown began. For many, amid so much unthinkable tragedy, the pandemic brought a newfound appreciation for what their bodies could do, beyond how their bodies looked.

Women's desire to test their strength and endurance through exercise is now widely accepted in this country. But until relatively recently, the premise that an average woman would regularly break a sweat in the name of health—or even beauty or weight loss— would have shocked most Americans.

Throughout the first half of the twentieth century, sweating was considered unladylike, and women tried to hide their muscles under sleeves. While women's beauty guides advised that gentle calisthenics could help correct a woman's "figure faults," doctors cautioned against vigorous exercise, warning it would lead to exhaustion or make a woman's uterus literally fall out. Until the early 1970s, common wisdom held it was dangerous for women to run more than a couple of miles at a time—a justification for banning women from road races. The average woman exercised so little for so long, the sports bra wasn't invented until 1977. (All hail inventors Lisa Lindahl, Hinda Miller, and Polly Smith.)

But while much has been written about how the rise of women's sports has empowered women, the role of women's *fitness* in shaping our collective pursuit of strength has largely slipped under the historical radar. This, despite the fact that most women stop playing organized sports when they graduate from high school or college, whereas many exercise for a lifetime.

When popular media have explored the historical significance of women's fitness culture, they have mostly treated it as a collection of disparate fads with little impact on women's lives or society at large. It is often covered as kitsch—reminders of a past that women would just as soon forget, from vibrating belts that promised to eviscerate fat to neon leg warmers.

We can always find reasons to laugh at the choices made by our younger, less wise selves or forebearers—*thong* leotards? really?—but this popular treatment also surely stems from the fact that we live in a culture that diminishes women's interests as silly and trivial. Dismissing the things women say they love as inconsequential allows our culture to stealthily ensure women remain subordinate to men.

American women's fitness history is more than a series of misguided "crazes." It's the story of how women have chosen to spend a collective billions of dollars and hours in pursuit of health and happiness. In many ways, it's the story of what it has meant to be a woman over the past seven decades.

For much of the twentieth century, most women didn't *move* very much. They grew up being told they were physically limited. "For centuries women have been shackled to a perception of themselves as weak and ineffectual," Colette Dowling writes in *The Frailty Myth*. "This perception has been nothing less than the emotional and cognitive equivalent of having our whole bodies bound."

By the late sixties, however, women began to question whether they really *were* defined by their biology. A new wave of feminists wondered: What if women weren't born physically weak, but became weak in a kind of self-fulfilling prophecy? After all, little boys were encouraged to climb trees and throw balls, while little girls were rewarded for displaying poise and grace. Boys were encouraged to get dirty; girls, to keep their clothes pristine. Even clothes themselves discouraged movement: The restrictive dresses, girdles, and high heels of mid-century women's wardrobes made it difficult for them to bend, stretch, run, and sometimes even breathe.

Men enjoyed a lifetime of practicing how to use and trust their bodies; women did not.

In the early seventies, the authors of the seminal women's health guide *Our Bodies, Ourselves* wrote: "Our bodies are the physical bases from which we move out into the world," but "ignorance, uncertainty—even, at worst, shame—about our physical selves create in us an alienation from ourselves that keeps us from being the whole people that we could be. Picture a woman trying to do work and to enter into equal and satisfying relationships with other people . . . when she feels physically weak because she has never tried to be strong."

The rise of women's fitness offered a path to this strength.

For most of her life, the feminist icon Gloria Steinem actively avoided exercise, feeling more comfortable living in her head. "I come from a generation who didn't do sports. Being a cheerleader or drum majorette was as far as our imaginations or role models could take us," she wrote in her book *Moving Beyond Words*. "That's one of many reasons why I and other women of my generation grew up believing—as many girls still do—that the most important thing about a female body is not what it does but how it looks. The power lies not within us but in the gaze of the observer."

As she watched friends begin to exercise in the seventies and eighties, her perspective shifted. "For women to enjoy physical strength is a collective revolution," Steinem later wrote. "I've gradually come to believe that society's acceptance of muscular women may be one of the most intimate, visceral measures of change," she also observed. "Yes, we need progress everywhere, but an increase in our physical strength could have more impact on the everyday lives of most women than the occasional role model in the boardroom or in the White House."

Steinem herself began practicing yoga and lifting weights in her fifties.

Of course, women's fitness culture is far from universally empowering. As this book will make clear, it is deeply intertwined with beauty culture, which sells the idea that women must change to be lovable—or even acceptable. Over the decades, fitness purveyors promising to lift women up have instead held them back and held them down by exploiting their insecurities. And the fitness industry at large is a formidable capitalist force that has long tried to commodify women's empowerment for its own gain. But to dismiss the rise of women's fitness culture as *only* harmful is to deny the experiences of millions who consider exercise vital to their well-being. Put simply: It's a lot more nuanced than good or bad.

Like my experience with Pure Barre, many women start exercising to change their appearance, but they stick with it after discovering more meaningful rewards. For some, becoming strong helps them overcome the desire to shape their body for anyone else's pleasure. As journalist Haley Shapley writes in *Strong Like Her*, "strength begets strength," and not just of the muscular variety.

By understanding women's fitness history—the good *and* the bad, the silly *and* the serious—we can better understand ourselves. And we can better harness exercise in ways that truly liberate all women.

My own fitness history began nearly four decades ago. I grew up in Atlanta in the eighties and nineties, the era of Get in Shape, Girl! toy sets and Great Shape Barbie—who came equipped with a teal spandex catsuit, leg warmers, and heels that never touched the ground— and later, the ThighMaster and *Buns of Steel* home video series.

While I knew early on that exercise was "good for you," I mainly thought of it as a ticket to becoming thin and conventionally attractive. I was average-sized as a teenager, but I believed that once I became a leaner me, through conviction and discipline, I would be a better me. A fully realized me. Like so many ambitious girls, I wanted to be big and small at the same time—to live a big life in a small body.

From middle school through my twenties, I saw exercise more as a chore, a female duty, than as a fun and invigorating way to spend my time. I saw my body—my arms, abs, thighs, and "buns"—as parts that needed to be mastered, Suzanne Somers style. I hoped I could jog and crunch and squat my way to perfection.

As I entered my thirties, exercise began to play a more profound role in my life. My dad is a lifelong runner, and his enthusiasm for the sport is contagious. I had always liked running, but running toward a "bikini body" took some of the joy out of it. When I stopped focusing on how running might transform my appearance, I began to enjoy the experience itself. Since turning thirty, I've run a dozen half-marathons and one full marathon, and I consider the sport core to my identity. I've taken cardio dance classes and felt the ecstasy of losing myself in the music. Barre classes, it turned out, offered me my first real taste of full-body muscular strength.

But it wasn't until I became pregnant, at thirty-six, that I began to truly appreciate the value of movement and strength. During most of my pregnancy, I felt powerful knowing I was growing a new life inside me. But after my son was born, I felt diminished. I'd endured a third-trimester blood pressure spike and an emergency C-section. For the first time, I didn't trust my body. For weeks that turned into months after giving birth, consumed by caring for a newborn, my husband and I rarely left home, and usually only to shuffle to the drugstore for diapers. Over time, the muscles I'd cultivated from running and barre became soft. My legs became tired. When I tried to locate my abs, I couldn't find them. I don't mean in the mirror. Standing in my bedroom one morning with my breast-milk-stained Gap sleep shirt raised, my son already a few months old, I poked and pressed, attempting to flex and feel at least a remnant of resistance. Instead, I felt only a void.

But I didn't want my pre-baby body "back." I didn't feel like the person I was before I gave birth, and trying to re-create her felt like going backward. Yet I did want to feel in control again, to feel strong again. Strong enough to nurture a baby and marriage and career. The pursuit of physical power now felt urgent. When I was ready to start exercising again, doctors, family members—everyone who cared about me—cheered me on.

While writing this book, I learned how fortunate I am to be living in an era when women are encouraged to move. But I also gained deeper insight into the reality that because of systemic inequality and discrimination, exercise is not a right but a privilege in this country. The fitness industry has a history of exclusion, catering to middle- and upper-class white people with disposable income. The costs associated with working out make it inaccessible to millions. Exercise also requires time and a safe space to move around in—luxuries millions more don't have. Just as the rich often get richer, the fit often get fitter, while the poor get sicker. And then there's the problematic fact that exercising has, for several decades, been linked to virtue, creating stigmas against people who can't or don't want to or even don't *look like* they work out.

Examining how and why these injustices came to be—and spreading awareness—can help to make fitness more inclusive of and accessible to all women. There are signs of progress, as a new generation of pioneers is dedicating their lives to this goal.

———————

This book tells the story of how America transformed from a nation where women saw vigorous exercise as "unfeminine" to the world we live in today, where so many consider physical activity a way of life. It reveals how the pursuit of fitness and beauty became so intertwined. And most of all, it showcases the pioneers who, through each era of this country's history, fought for women's right to move. These trailblazers—inspiring, outspoken, complicated women—shaped the substance and rhythm of women's daily lives and laid the groundwork for today's fitness landscape. While they were media sensations in their day, "viral" before viral was a thing, most have been overlooked by popular histories.

Our story begins in the fifties, when the first real women's fitness celebrity, Bonnie Prudden, pitched exercise as a novel solution for housewives who felt trapped in their homes and struggled to find purpose outside their roles as wives and mothers. We'll travel to London in the Swinging Sixties, when miniskirts and the brewing sexual revolution helped to fuel Lotte Berk's barre classes.

From there, we'll see how, in the seventies, women found liberation through jogging, and how Jazzercise and aerobic dancing became American institutions. We'll trace Jane Fonda's extraordinary path from film ingenue and anti–Vietnam War activist to Hollywood's first celebrity fitness influencer.

We'll explore why women started lifting weights and eventually wanted "buns of steel"—and why, after years of striving for hard bodies at the gym, they turned to yoga by the tens of millions. Finally, we'll look at the new vanguard of women's fitness pioneers, embodied by Instagram and yoga superstar Jessamyn Stanley, who are working to bring exercise to every body.

I hope you find this history as engrossing to read as it was to research—a journey that included interviewing bona fide fitness legends, scouring more than seven decades of fitness books, poring through archival women's magazines, sweating to home workout tapes, and speaking with dozens of exercise enthusiasts who ran, danced, lifted, tucked, and stretched through the events in these pages. And I hope, like me, you will find that understanding how and why we move can help us better understand ourselves.

All right, ladies. Are you ready? Let's go.

CHAPTER 1

Reduce

Pat: I've been around physical ed for years.
Mike: Physical Ed? Who's he?

—Katharine Hepburn and Spencer Tracy
in *Pat and Mike*, 1952

America, manpower conscious, is almost oblivious
of the potential of its neglected womanpower.

—Eugene *Register-Guard*, 1962

N ew Yorkers who spotted Bonnie Prudden striding through midtown Manhattan in August 1957 couldn't have known they were glimpsing the future. With the space race revving up and new technological marvels emerging every day—color TV! Teflon pans!—who would give serious consideration to a petite forty-something woman going about her day in a stretchy jumpsuit? She was an anomaly, a head-scratcher. They couldn't have known that someday their city would be filled with Bonnies, sheathed in work-out clothes that allowed them to move as they pleased.

But that summer, after weekly appearances on NBC's *Home* show, she knew she was onto something. The morning show was hosted by Arlene Francis and Hugh Downs, and featured her, America's leading fitness expert, alongside some of the biggest names of the day—Bob Hope, Jerry Lewis, Dear Abby's Abigail Van Buren. "We are raising a nation of children with muscles of custard," Bonnie told the hosts. She had a gift for dramatic exaggeration that annoyed her critics. The whole *country* was falling apart, she said.

Now the editors at *Sports Illustrated* seemed to agree, asking her to appear on the cover of their August 5 issue as both a model of physical fitness and its number one champion. So what if they'd be featuring her during the languid final stretch of summer? A cover was a cover.

It would be the latest in a string of platforms to promote her controversial message: Everyone should exercise. *Everyone.* Every day. Even the mostly male readers of a magazine devoted largely to golf and baseball highlights—who thumbed through issues while smoking cigarettes and sipping scotch, or grabbing 25-cent burgers at a coffee shop counter on a lunch break, only to commute via train or bus or car home, where they would plop into an easy chair and watch a few hours of television. Even their girlfriends and wives, who were raised to believe ladies should never sweat. (*Horses sweat, men perspire, but ladies merely glow*, went the old adage.)

For the cover, shot at her "fitness institute" in the suburb of White Plains—a predecessor to the kind of gyms that would become a fixture in this country decades later—Bonnie slipped into her trademark workout uniform, a one-piece wool outfit of her own design called a "leotite," covered in a jaunty star pattern.

It was a novel concept, both the outfit and the notion that a woman would prioritize comfort and flexibility in her wardrobe. After all, it was a moment when most of the decade's fashions were shaped by girdles and petticoats. Once, when Bonnie was late to an appointment, she ran through the streets of Manhattan in one of her leotites covered only by a thin white medical coat. A well-meaning police officer stopped her—*Was she okay?* he wanted to know. It was highly unusual for a woman to be running in public, and especially one so scantily clad.

Sports Illustrated assigned staff photographer Richard Meek, whose previous credits included baseball great Ted Williams and hockey legend Gordie Howe, to her cover shoot. Bonnie styled her close-cropped brown curls into a no-fuss 'do and wore just a smidge of makeup. Her leotite advertised that her arms, legs, stomach— every inch of her 5-foot-3-inch frame—were harder than those of most women her age (or any age). Her boundless energy belied her forty-three years, the challenges of raising two teen daughters, her chronic loneliness.

For the winning photo, Bonnie got down on the ground, shot a toned leg high into the air, and smiled. *Click!* The move was so familiar to her, but so exotic to most Americans. Inside the magazine, the reading line accompanying her feature would offer this mantra: *Bonnie Prudden says: You are NOT too young, too old, too full of aches, too fat, too thin, too far gone, too lazy, too flabby, too anything to have fun keeping fit.* She would devote the next few pages attempting to convince a skeptical nation.

"The secret is simple," she told readers. You "substitute activity for inactivity as much as you can during the course of a normal day and take a few minutes of each day to do some easy exercises." It was straightforward enough. "For more fun and best results do the exercises to music," she added. "Use Leroy Anderson's 'Sleigh Ride' or 'China Doll.'" Women should "never wear girdles while exercising," she warned, "but *should* wear a brassiere."

She demonstrated four floor exercises to get readers started, the first in a pictorial column that would run in more than forty issues of the magazine.

The secret may have been simple, but it was a tough sell in postwar America. What would daily exercise look like for Americans in the late fifties? For men, it would mean reconsidering the three-martini lunch. For women, it would mean something more profound: taking time out of their day to care for themselves, when nearly every social institution stressed that a woman's sole purpose in life was to care for others.

Unless exercise could be sold as a wifely duty—and a path to winning the Cold War.

Americans had long prided themselves on being a hardy people. They were puritans and pioneers and immigrants, tough and industrious. They were can-do workers and strivers. But by the 1950s, they were moving less than ever before, and the lack of activity was taking a toll. Politicians and pundits questioned whether the nation was becoming soft.

Gone were the days when Americans' survival depended on physical competence. As the twentieth century progressed, the growing middle class embraced what it called "our modern way of life." It was a lifestyle defined by ease and abundance, which felt like a balm after the Great Depression and World War II. It prized comfort, convenience, efficiency. It also made Americans' bodies "largely irrelevant," writes historian Shelly McKenzie in *Getting Physical: The Rise of Fitness Culture in America*.

The rise of the suburbs transformed nearly every aspect of middle-class life, as a single-family home with a yard in a well-groomed neighborhood became the new American dream. From 1950 to 1960, the country's suburban population exploded from 21 million to 37 million. But over time, those living in the new sprawl succumbed to what Bonnie Prudden liked to call "the tyranny of the wheel." Walking was replaced by driving, as cars were now required to get around. Kids who in previous generations had been active since they could scoot were now pushed in strollers, then shuttled to school in buses. (No more walking a mile, uphill both ways, in the snow, to class.) Children also had fewer open spaces for playing and fewer trees for climbing, as land was paved into parking lots. In many towns sidewalks were narrowed or eliminated completely.

Suburban homes themselves were built and furnished to minimize physical exertion. The decade's popular one-story ranch houses eliminated the need to climb stairs. Air-conditioning units and central heating and new push-button appliances required only the touch of a finger. By 1960, three-quarters of families owned cars and washing machines, and 90 percent owned a television, as sitting in front of the small screen became a favorite American pastime.

Women still did plenty of housework, of course—a woman's work truly was never done—but as anyone who has ever cleaned a home knows, the physical labor it requires doesn't always benefit the body. Bonnie Prudden warned as much. "Housework won't raise a bosom to where it belongs or keep it there," she told a reporter in 1956. "Housework is no good for all-round muscular fitness."

Then there was the matter of the dinner table. Americans were eating more, and they were eating *worse*. In the fifties, the "golden age of food processing," the food industry churned out mass quantities of products rich in sugar, salt, fat, and preservatives. The decade saw the birth of McDonald's, Burger King, Kentucky Fried Chicken, and Dunkin' Donuts. Swanson introduced the "TV dinner" to the masses in 1954, after the company found itself with a surplus of 260 tons of turkey after Thanksgiving, and it sold 10 million in the first year. Supermarkets expanded to house the vast quantities of new, modern cuisine. As Cold War fears grew, the government drilled home the message that democracy was defined by abundance—and communism by scarcity—which turned purchasing into a patriotic act. Madison Avenue admen and -women reinforced these values by linking factory-made food with positive emotions: family, celebration, and love.

When Americans went to work, they sat some more, as desk jobs surged. In many professions, drinking on the job was accepted or encouraged, and considered a necessary lubricant to woo clients and conduct daily business. (The Time & Life Building that housed *Sports Illustrated* offered staff a dimly lit room where employees could lie down during the day if they overdid it at lunch.) Factory jobs didn't involve as much sitting or imbibing, but they did become more automated.

To top it all off, more Americans were smoking more cigarettes, too. Smoking had gradually increased throughout the century largely thanks to Hollywood, which portrayed cigarettes as sexy, sophisticated, and glamorous. By 1964, when the U.S. Surgeon General first revealed cigarettes could cause lung and laryngeal cancers, 40 percent of adults smoked—not to mention hordes of teen baby boomers.

The "modern way of life" was starting to impact American bodies. While the rise of vaccines and antibiotics had dramatically lowered rates of contagious and infectious diseases, the country now saw a surge in disease borne out of abundance. More Americans began to suffer from hypertension, diabetes, gallbladder disease, and heart attacks. Meanwhile, military generals reported that new recruits were weak, raising fears about America's ability to defend itself. During World War I, the military turned down 37 percent of potential draftees for being physically unfit; by the Korean War, it rejected 52 percent. As Bonnie Prudden was discovering through her own research, even the country's kids had grown weaker and less limber.

But few Americans saw exercise as the solution.

Mid-century Americans loathed exercise. They considered it painfully boring, a silly way to spend one's precious leisure time.

"The mere mention of formal exercise is enough to bring a shudder to the average American spine, weak as it is alleged to be at present," Robert H. Boyle wrote in *Sports Illustrated* in 1955. Besides, few medical experts were telling people they *should* exercise. Doctors were more concerned about the dangers of over-exertion than under-exertion, believing strenuous exercise could lead to heart attacks in men and reproductive problems in women. "Whenever I get the urge to exercise, I lie down until the feeling passes," University of Chicago president Robert Maynard Hutchins famously quipped, and in the 1950s, he spoke for the mainstream.

Mid-century Americans with the time and means played sports and games, to be sure—tennis and golf, sailing and skiing. Young men played baseball, basketball, and football; young women rode horses, danced, or played volleyball or field hockey or half-court basketball in knee-length skirts. Some people swam, if they had access to a pool. Americans might accidentally break a sweat dancing the jitterbug or hula-hooping. And a few "kept fit" by doing calisthenics—a nineteenth-century term that comes from the Greek for beautiful strength—recognizing that stretching and moving their bodies made them feel good. But for most, exercise was the by-product of sport, not an activity unto itself. Few saw the point of exercising to maintain one's health or quality of life. There was no such thing as training, unless you were an athlete preparing for competition.

American popular culture treated those who did devote significant time to exercising—and particularly to building muscle—as oddities, or worse. Thanks partly to Hollywood's portrayal of muscular men as thickheaded, the public generally believed that brain and brawn were incompatible. Men with big, visible muscles were often cast as villainous henchmen, thugs, or simply dummies. In other cases, men who appeared overly concerned with their physique were viewed with suspicion. In a culture that was deeply homophobic, such behavior was thought to signal homosexuality.

Americans would learn, in time, the power of daily movement. But the summer Bonnie Prudden posed for her *Sports Illustrated* cover, her suggestion that Americans—men, women, and children—make a regular habit of exercising and strengthening their bodies struck most as ridiculous.

During a 1956 radio interview with journalist Mike Wallace, the future *60 Minutes* correspondent asks Bonnie, with a chuckle: "You think that there should be a formal exercise, a kind of 'joy through strength' period for husband, wife, and family when the father gets home from work at six thirty at night, before the martinis? . . . You think that we should have a routine, *all* of us?" To which she responds without missing a beat: "I'm more convinced of it than you are." For a country bracing for a war against the Soviets, however, becoming a nation of "softies" wasn't acceptable, either. The lady in the leotite was offering a solution.

———————

Ruth "Bonnie" Prudden was a descendant of Davy Crockett, the folk hero crowned "King of the Wild Frontier," and she wore her lineage like a badge of honor.

She had been hyperactive as a kid. She never walked anywhere, she liked to say—she ran. In 1918, when she was four years old, she began a habit of climbing out of a second-story window of her family's home at midnight and roaming the streets of their middle-class neighborhood in Mount Vernon, just north of the Bronx. Her father was concerned and suggested her mother take her to the family doctor. *Why so much energy?* she asked the doctor.

"There is nothing wrong with this child that discipline and exhaustion won't cure," the doctor said. He suggested they enroll Bonnie in a local Russian ballet academy, and it worked. "After my three strenuous dance classes each week, I was much too tired to wander in the night." Her parents would soon supplement her dancing with classes at German and Swedish gymnastics schools as well.

As she grew up, Bonnie became a "scrubby little tomboy." She went bare-legged in the New York winters, her knees covered in cuts and bruises from climbing, exploring, adventuring. "When I wanted to find out if I liked a boy, I'd climb a tree and challenge him to follow me," she would say. "If he couldn't make it, he was out."

Bonnie's life indoors was lonely. Her mother's worsening alcoholism and sharp tongue created constant stress. She could feel her mother's disappointment in having birthed such an aberrant daughter. "I was not frail, not pretty, nor golden haired and blue-eyed. That was my little sister, Jeanne," Bonnie wrote. "My mother's repetitive question, *Why can't you be more like your sister?*, was a thorn in my heart." Bonnie preferred spending time with her father, who was an outdoorsman, but he worked in newspaper advertising and was rarely home. When he was, he liked to call his eldest daughter his "bonnie lass"—a nickname that stuck.

Bonnie loved to read, to be transported to other worlds through books, but her talent for dance would be the thing that would grant her access to real-life new worlds. After graduating in 1933 from New York City's Horace Mann School, she spent a summer working at a ranch in Arizona, where her "well-trained body learned to break horses, brand and castrate cattle, and ride for days." She returned to New York that fall and took a few college courses before joining a professional dance company. Bonnie loved performing; her mother wondered aloud what would become of her daughter. At twenty-one, she snagged her dream job—a role dancing in a Broadway musical revue called *Life Begins at 8:40*.

A year after joining the show, Bonnie married the man she had been dating since high school, an aspiring artist and Dartmouth grad named Dick Hirschland. Dick's father had emigrated from Germany to America before his country descended into fascism. In their sprawling estate in the tony Westchester suburb of Harrison, his parents ran a kind of way station for German Jews seeking refuge, hosting them until they found their footing.

The elder Hirschlands believed their son and his new wife should live a conventional life. Dick wanted to be a professional artist, but his parents felt their family was better suited to collecting than creating art, and arranged for him to take over a hundred-thousand-dollar manufacturing business "on its last legs." Nor did they approve of Bonnie's career. Her father-in-law "would not have a professional dancer in the family" and forced her to abruptly quit the show. Her place was in the home, her in-laws told her. The newlyweds set about forging a life neither of them wanted.

Still, for a while, they were happy together. Dick loved to ski and rock climb (he aced Bonnie's tree-climbing test), and he encouraged Bonnie to join him on trips to the mountains. She showed an immediate talent for both sports. On their honeymoon to Europe, the couple climbed the famed Swiss-Italian Matterhorn. They spent many weekends ascending the Shawangunks, affectionately known as the Gunks, a mountain range about eighty miles north of New York City. They spent others descending ski slopes.

Before long, Bonnie became a star in both the climbing and skiing worlds. She would later have a Gunks cliff named after her, when she became the first person to ascend a difficult climb now known as Bonnie's Roof. She would also become a member of the Westchester ski patrol and the first woman to earn a safety award from the Eastern Amateur Ski Association. But the higher she climbed, the lower she felt at home.

Not long into their marriage, Bonnie suffered a skiing accident that would mark the beginning of the end of her relationship with Dick and the start of the rest of her life. While flying down a trail at the Suicide Six ski resort near Woodstock, Vermont, she crashed into a rock and fractured her pelvis in four places. Her doctor told her she would always walk with a limp and never ski or climb or dance again, nor have children. She was determined to prove him wrong. She had developed an intimate trust of her body through her years as an athlete. *Come on,* her body whispered to her. *You've been busted before. You'll be okay.*

One day, when Bonnie was finally able to sit up in bed, her nurse put on a record of the fast-paced "Dipsy Doodle." "Quite without any conscious direction from me, my feet started tapping," she later wrote. She saw an opportunity. "In half an hour I had choreographed a foot and leg routine that felt wonderful. I was in a lather and needed a nap." That afternoon she choreographed another "bed ballet."

In the Gunks she'd met Dr. Hans Kraus, a renowned climber and orthopedist who trained in Vienna, and who would later become one of President John F. Kennedy's White House personal physicians. At the time, Dr. Kraus worked at Columbia-Presbyterian Hospital's Back Clinic. Could he help? He prescribed her a series of exercises, and through her recovery, she discovered the benefits of daily stretching and strengthening. She began to wonder: *Why didn't more people exercise* before *getting injured, as well as after?*

She got rid of her limp, started dancing again, and returned to the cliffs and slopes.

She also got pregnant.

———————

Despite their excursions to the mountains, Bonnie feared her marriage to Dick was deteriorating. Dick was miserable in the career his father chose for him, and the misery seeped through to their relationship. Her skiing accident sent him further into a funk. When Bonnie told her husband he was becoming a father, he responded with: "Now you've spoiled everything." How could they go to the mountains with a baby?

In 1939, Bonnie gave birth to their first daughter, Joan, and four years later a second daughter, Susan. Becoming a mother did not, as Dick had moaned, stop her from mountaineering. She raised her daughters to be as active as she was, teaching them to swim, ski, ride horses, dance, even climb: By six years old, both daughters had ascended two mountains.

Bonnie's aspirations for her daughters would ultimately reshape the trajectory of her own life—and that of the nation. One fateful day when Joan was in the third grade, Bonnie decided to visit her daughter's PE class at her public school in the Westchester suburb of Harrison. Bonnie had loved PE as a little girl, where she had learned marching and the Virginia reel. But now she watched, "horrified," she later recounted, as a teacher in skirts and heels guided twenty-five little girls through circle games for twenty minutes. There was nothing physical about her daughter's physical education.

Bonnie would pace a room while she thought or spoke, and she was surely pacing that night. She couldn't stop thinking about what she'd observed. *That's it*, she decided. She would start teaching her own physical education classes, the way phys ed ought to be taught. She would happily teach whatever kids were interested for free. She didn't want another child to miss out on the joys of feeling physically competent.

Bonnie managed to recruit twelve neighborhood children—five girls and seven boys—to exercise after school. The girls' moms balked at the suggestion, saying they didn't want their daughters to "get muscles." But Bonnie was persuasive, and she confidently told them, as she would later tell millions, that "under every curve is a muscle. No muscle, no curve."* The parents of other kids politely declined—they couldn't fathom making their children exercise.

Bonnie quickly rebranded, clarifying that she was teaching

---

* Not exactly true, but a savvy sales pitch at the time.

"conditioning." More parents bought it. "No one had a preconceived idea of what that word meant."

In six weeks, she had attracted dozens of neighborhood kids, then double and triple that. She used "wild and woolly music," working hard to make the classes fun. "I got them to run and jump and do all the things any child will naturally do if given a chance." Local schools let her use their gyms, as long as she agreed to teach any child who showed up.

After a while, Bonnie wanted a way to track her students' progress. She again consulted Dr. Hans Kraus, this time while the two rested on a ledge thousands of feet high in the mountains. *What did he advise?* Kraus told her about a strength and flexibility test he had developed with another physician at his clinic, Dr. Sonja Weber. The test included six simple exercises for evaluating the abdominal and lower back muscles, including sit-ups and bending over to touch one's toes. But, he explained, it was designed for patients struggling with back and posture disabilities. Healthy children would pass easily.

Bonnie decided to administer the so-called Kraus-Weber Test anyway.

Not long into her testing, she couldn't believe what she was seeing: More than half of her new students failed. However, among her more experienced and "conditioned" students, only 8 percent failed.

Kraus was astounded. "Can you test the whole town?" he asked.

Bonnie jumped at the assignment.

By the early 1950s, Bonnie and Hans had grown close. They climbed together—Hans was feet behind her when she ascended Bonnie's Roof—supporting each other through adrenaline-pumping feats. Hans was handsome, rugged, smart, and successful; he loved women, and women loved him. With Bonnie's marriage crumbling, they began an affair she knew was not destined to last, but that provided her with at least a modicum of the love and affection she craved.

"We fell in love," she later wrote in her journal, "and I'm sure he was by far the more surprised. He had had so many loves . . . there must have been hundreds. I was just another admiring woman . . . one who liked to listen to him . . . in whose eyes he too saw a mirror."

Their professional affair would lead to more lasting rewards.

Around this time Hans joined the staff of New York University's Institute of Physical Medicine and Rehabilitation, and Bonnie officially became his research assistant. For seven years, "I tested anyone I could get my hands on between the ages of six and sixteen," she wrote. This added up to more than 7,000 youngsters across the United States and half a dozen countries around the world.

In America, Hans and Bonnie found that young people consistently failed the fitness test at a rate of 58 percent, with urban kids performing slightly worse than their suburban and rural counterparts. But what they observed in Europe blew their minds all over again. During climbing expeditions abroad, they carved out time to test local children, and they soon discovered that kids in Italy, Austria, and Switzerland—for whom movement was still a big part of their daily life—scored significantly better than Americans: Their failure rate was only 9 percent.

What were the implications of the physical weakness of American kids? Hans and Bonnie dubbed the condition hypokinetic disease, meaning disease due to lack of movement. Their research revealed an increased risk of coronary heart disease, diabetes, duodenal ulcer, muscle tension, low back pain, and "psychiatric problems." They compiled their findings in a paper titled "Hypokinetic Disease: Role of Inactivity in Production of Disease" and later published it in *The New York State Journal of Medicine*.

The world took notice slowly at first. *Ladies' Home Journal*, which reached a staggering 15 million readers, covered their findings in March 1954, in a feature headlined, "How Fit Are Our Children?"

It teased: "School buses, television, sports for the few—these are part of America's way of life. But what do they mean to our children's health?" Other magazines and newspapers asked, "Is your child a 'softie'?"

A growing minority were becoming alarmed. But for a while, life went on as usual for Bonnie, and she turned her attention back to spreading her fitness gospel at home.

Bonnie had been teaching conditioning classes for six years, and she was itching to go bigger. When she learned about an abandoned two-story elementary school for sale in nearby White Plains, New York, she saw her chance—father-in-law be damned.

In 1953, she purchased the "gloomy old school" and gutted it down to its "beautiful brick walls and shining eight-foot windows." She brought in reinforcing steel beams and painted the walls white and yellow. The polished hardwood floors were perfect for dance and calisthenics. She installed three large gymnasiums, two dance studios, a Finnish sauna, two massage rooms, a snack bar, locker rooms, and a massive Madison Avenue–style office for herself. She painted the equipment, "designed after the curbs, fences, railroad tracks of a less mechanized day," in bright colors. Outside, she installed an obstacle course that included America's first climbing wall, along with nets, hurdles, parallel bars, ladders, ramps, a maze, and a tightrope.

Bonnie opened for business in 1954, calling her school the Institute for Physical Fitness. In an advertisement announcing its opening, she promised to build "strong, flexible, attractive bodies" and raise "the fitness level of all." (The ad noted the school was "especially equipped to handle 'teen-age Awkwardness.'") Bonnie's potent combination of respectability and swagger was enough to convince dubious suburbanites to come and see for themselves.

That same year, she flew to Reno and divorced Dick Hirschland.

Nearly a year after Hans and Bonnie published their report, an article about their findings would make its way to John B. Kelly Sr., a wealthy Philadelphia contractor and former Olympic sculler (and, incidentally, the father of actress Grace Kelly). He was appalled, and he shared the report with a senator friend from Pennsylvania. The senator, James H. Duff, brought it all the way to the Oval Office.

President Dwight Eisenhower was already concerned about the nation's fitness. He had emerged as a national hero after serving as a five-star general during World War II and was disturbed by the fact that half of America's men had been declared unfit to serve. He had also begun to worry that, with the rise of professional sports, too many kids (boys) were developing "spectatoritis"—watching others be active instead of being active themselves. The report set off alarm bells. The president would host a summit at the White House to discuss its findings.

On a balmy July 11, 1955, Bonnie, then forty-one years old, arrived at 1600 Pennsylvania Avenue wearing a borrowed hat and dark suit. She was nervous, scared "spitless." As she looked around the luncheon, she saw what *Sports Illustrated* would call "the greatest array of U.S. sport stars ever gathered together in one place." There was baseball luminary Willie Mays and basketball phenom Bill Russell. There were golf stars, and the president of the Boy Scouts of America. She was glad to see John B. Kelly Sr., without whom none of them would be there. The only other woman invited was a golfer named Barbara Romack.

The president and his guests took their seats, and it was time for Hans and Bonnie to present their research. When Bonnie glanced at the president, he smiled warmly, and she relaxed. They talked the room through their findings, underscoring how poorly American youngsters fared and the potential long-term effects of the modern way of life.

The president took it all in, then responded: He was *stunned.* Something had to be done.

After the luncheon, a breathless media dubbed Hans's and Bonnie's findings "The Report That Shocked the President" and dubbed Bonnie the "gym teacher to the nation's children." Reporters from New York to Los Angeles began contacting her at the institute. It wasn't just the nation's children who were in trouble, she would say. "I don't see this country lasting 30 years unless we get on the ball right away," she told one journalist. "We were once the greatest nation, today we're the weakest in the world. We've taken the physical life out of America."

The report was not without its critics. In an angry letter to the president, one Democratic congressman wrote: "According to Dr. Kraus' statement, the physical fitness of American children is eight times lower than the physical fitness of European children. Simply on the mathematical surface, this is a ridiculous statement, and I am very much surprised that you would dignify it." Two physical education graduate students at Iowa State University who were initially interested in administering the Kraus-Weber Test themselves spoke out about what they viewed as a major flaw. In order to "pass," participants had to pass all six exercises. Failing even one of the six meant they "failed" the entire test, which didn't seem accurate. Indeed, the bar was high.

But many physical education leaders applauded them, and the president vowed to create a special council to improve the fitness of the nation's kids. He gave the task of creating the President's Council on Youth Fitness to his vice president, Richard Nixon.* The White House would host a bigger fitness summit in late September 1955 at

---

* Remember those stress-inducing (if you were me) Presidential Physical Fitness Tests you might have had to undergo twice a year in PE class as a kid? The "shuttle run" and the "sit-and-reach"? Yes, you can thank Bonnie Prudden.

an Air Force base in Denver, bringing together more than a hundred physical education, medical, and sports figures. Days before the gathering, however, President Eisenhower suffered a heart attack on a nearby golf course. His medical emergency spooked the country and seemed to confirm that America was suffering from a "cardiac crisis." If the larger-than-life Army general was vulnerable, anyone was at risk.

The Denver summit was held as planned, followed by another summit the following year in Annapolis, Maryland. Bonnie attended both, but after the initial high of the White House luncheon, she felt discouraged. The problem of the nation's fitness could not, it seemed to her, be solved by committee. The more so-called experts they brought in to address the problem, the murkier the solution became.

"Talk talk talk," Bonnie told *Sports Illustrated* of the efforts. "The country is disappearing while we sit around and talk about it. It's like the story somebody told me of the people who argued about which fire hydrant to use while the church burned down."

After "The Report That Shocked the President," Bonnie became a star—her name synonymous with health, fitness, and, perhaps most crucial, attractiveness. Where the county's elected leaders were vague about how to be fit, Bonnie was specific and direct. Publishing houses invited Bonnie to write books detailing her regimens, and she churned out one guide after another: *Is Your Child Really Fit?* in 1956 and *Bonnie Prudden's Fitness Book* in 1959. She made an exercise record, *Keep Fit / Be Happy with Bonnie Prudden*, for families to follow in their living rooms. "Fitness should begin in the cradle," she would tell mothers, encouraging them to put away the playpens and let their kids run around to develop their muscles.

But it wasn't too late for mothers, either.

Bonnie's success convincing America that everyday women—girls, teens, mothers, and grandmothers—could benefit from regular exercise was perhaps her most extraordinary accomplishment. Its legacy, however, would have mixed consequences.

Bonnie had always thought of herself as being as capable as a man—more capable than many. She knew she was as talented as the men she skied and climbed with, and she didn't much consider her gender on the ropes or slopes. (Once, when she was climbing with Hans and another man, she told them: "Well, the time has come." She needed to pee. The men lowered her cord down six feet. She did what she had to do, then kept on climbing.) She believed to her core that men and women were equal. She told skeptical mothers again and again that girls and women could and *should* do push-ups, that strength and flexibility would allow girls to get the most out of life.

But Bonnie also knew the rewards of being physically attractive and the allure of physical transformation. And so, in the same breath in which she proselytized about the importance of women being strong, she also sold the power of exercise to shape, or reduce, one's figure.

When *Sports Illustrated* sent reporter Dorothy Stull to cover her Institute for Physical Fitness in 1956—a year before Bonnie would appear on the magazine's cover—Stull was struck by the number of women exercising inside and outside the facility. "Under Bonnie's magic spell, sophisticated suburban matrons delight in scaling mountainous walls," she writes. "And some of them, victims of A-bomb era tensions, discover for the first time the blissful euphoria of purely physical fatigue."

At one point during Stull's visit, Bonnie steps into her office dressing room to change out of the white collared blouse and tailored shorts she'd been wearing to exercise and slips into "a soft silk low-necked dress that clung to her figure." She leans in conspiratorially and offers Stull a cocktail from her bar cart.

"People think you shouldn't drink if you want to be a good example of fitness," Bonnie tells her, tossing her curls. "I say, the main reason for having a good body is to get the most out of life—and that means having fun, and it may mean having a drink now and then."

Later, she throws out a novel notion: "Every woman needs to be attractive, but to be so is not our due for being born, it is our reward for physical activity."

But what *could* fitness look like for women, when sweating was uncouth? When women's magazines told them to pretend they needed a man to open the pickle jar? To never beat a man in sports (or anything)? When it was illegal in some states for a woman to wear "men's clothing"? When many husbands had legal authority over their wife's body? In the years after World War II, it was unthinkable that an average woman would openly take up exercise to become strong. After all, nearly every social institution told her she should relinquish her power—for the sake of the country and the proper social order.

It hadn't always been this way for women. In the 1930s, as the country recovered from the Great Depression, women were encouraged to be physically capable—athletic, even. During the war, the government enlisted Rosies to be riveters, taking the place of men who had been called into combat. In the iconic war propaganda poster, Rosie's flexed (albeit small) muscle and her catchphrase, *We Can Do It!*, came to represent the nation's resilience. But after the war, as traumatized GIs returned home, the country's leaders told women to go home, too. "The war was over," wrote media scholar Susan J. Douglas in *Where the Girls Are: Growing Up Female with the Mass Media*, and women "were supposed to sashay back to the kitchen and learn how to make green beans baked with Campbell's cream of mushroom soup." By the end of the decade, more than half of the women who had been drawn into the workforce during the war relinquished (or were fired from) their jobs.

Women were told to "act like women" and "look like women," in part to fight the "paranoia that American women had become overly masculine during the war," writes historian Elizabeth Matelski in her book *Reducing Bodies: Mass Culture and the Female Figure in Postwar America*. They married earlier than their mothers had a generation ago, and they had more children in rapid succession.

Looking and acting like women did not include training for a marathon or lifting weights; femininity was defined by weakness.

Besides, for generations, doctors had warned that a woman who overexerted herself would suffer reproductive problems and never be able to have babies—which, for most women at the time, would have rendered them irrelevant. Girls grew up hearing they needed to take it very easy during their period—*for their own good*—and that too much exercise would cause their uterus to "fall out." (Bonnie liked to say, "I've observed hundreds of physical education classes around the world, and I have never seen a uterus on the gym floor.")

For girls who enjoyed being active—swimming or playing tennis or running around with the boys—they often hit a wall in middle or high school, when no organized sports were available to them. Girls in some areas could play basketball, but they could use only half the court—running the full court was believed to be too taxing. At many schools, girls' only formal outlets to be active were cheerleading and baton twirling. (It bears mentioning that cheerleading actually began as an exclusively male pursuit. Schools would select the most popular male students to rally up crowds with megaphones during games. It was only during World War II, when so many college men were drafted, that women began to replace them—a controversial move that some protested, fretting that for a girl to use her voice in such a way was unfeminine. When the men came back, they no longer wanted to participate in an activity that had been taken over by women.)

Young women who did have access and chose to devote

themselves to organized sports risked being labeled a jock. In an era when "acting like a woman" was code for "pleasing a man," being a jock was seen as deeply transgressive. It could also draw suspicions of lesbianism, deterring would-be athletes who didn't want their sexual orientation publicly examined.

Another barrier to women embracing vigorous exercise was the brewing Cold War and the prejudices it instilled against visibly muscular women. In the fifties, Soviet men and women alike participated in a rigorous national fitness program, creating a citizenship who was athletically impressive. And that effort paid off; in the 1960 Summer Olympics in Rome, the Soviets took home 103 medals to America's 71, prompting more national concern stateside. Americans perceived Russian women as powerful but mannish—*strong like bull.* As much as America wanted to beat the commies, it was equally important to American women that they be whatever Russian women weren't. "A fat, passive nation would be unable to compete with or combat Communism," writes Matelski. "But because Soviet women were active and strong, American women had to be the opposite."

But even as magazines and so-called experts encouraged women to hold themselves back emotionally, intellectually, and physically, they were also told they were never enough. "It is difficult for modern American women, steeped in the power of positive thinking, to realize how pervasive negative thinking was for women in the 1950s and early 1960s," writes historian Stephanie Coontz in her book *A Strange Stirring: The* Feminine Mystique *and American Women at the Dawn of the 1960s.* No one was telling women they could be whatever they wanted or do whatever they wanted; instead, women's magazines, which held enormous influence, continually told readers they should be doing *more, more, more* to be a better wife, mother, object of admiration.

"Women were encouraged to expect more than ever from marriage, but they were told that when a marriage fell short, it was almost invariably because they were not good enough wives," writes Coontz. "If a husband's bad behavior threatened the marriage, it was up to the wife to figure out what she had done to trigger this behavior and how she must change to bring out her husband's better side."

Naturally, one area women were constantly encouraged to improve was their appearance. The "marriage bargain" at the time included looking good for one's husband—a belief that led many a woman to never let her spouse see her without makeup, or to change from her daytime culottes into a freshly pressed dress before he arrived home from work, when she would greet him with a cocktail in hand. But it would take Bonnie Prudden and a handful of other fitness enthusiasts to sell the idea that vigorous physical activity could be a desirable path to beauty, grace, and sex appeal.

While the fitness industry was still in its early days, by the middle of the twentieth century the modern diet industry had exploded. Home scales became widely available, and magazines encouraged girls and women to keep close tabs on their weight and physical dimensions, propagating the notion that women needed to be thin to find and keep a man. Calorie counting became common practice. New fad diets emerged. Diet pill sales surged. Millions turned to cigarettes to suppress their appetite. Weight Watchers was founded in 1963. Even Disney's animated heroines had become slimmer, just as the country's population of teen girls ballooned—forming a massive, eager, deeply impressionable market for "reducing" advice and products.

America's Black communities had historically celebrated a wider range of sizes—historian Elizabeth Matelski cites a 1966 study suggesting that white teens were more concerned about weight loss than Black teens, even though the Black teens weighed more, and a fifth of Black teens actually wanted bigger hips and thighs. But in a country where white standards are all but enforced—the measures

against which culture and capitalism determine women's worth—
Black women also strove to be svelte.

And yet few women took up vigorous exercise to lose weight, both because such regimens would have been viewed as unfeminine and because doctors were just beginning to understand how exercise could lead to weight loss. In a 1953 Gallup poll, only 4 percent of dieters said they exercised. Their preferred methods for losing weight were diet pills, thyroid medication, and food restriction.

At a time when popular culture welcomed any technology that promised to make life easier, some women sought out so-called passive exercise at newly popular figure salons, also known as reducing salons, where they would hook themselves up to machines that promised to shake, roll, and pound away perceived figure flaws. (If technology could beam Ed Sullivan into their living room every week, why *couldn't* it eliminate flab?) "Although reducing salons were not health clubs per se, they helped entrench the habit of visiting a location outside the home for the improvement of one's body," writes historian Shelly McKenzie. "Figure salons appealed to women who wanted to shape their bodies but found exercise distasteful."

Among the most successful of these salons was a chain called Slenderella, whose ads vowed to slim women "in all the right places" without the "toil and suffering" of physical exertion. "While soft music played in the background, vibrating flat leather couches massaged patrons," writes historian Elizabeth Matelski. "The company claimed one forty-minute session at two dollars equaled a ten-mile horse ride or thirty-six holes of golf, and that afterward one's shoulders would be straightened, waistline slimmed, and muscles toned and firmed, with improved circulation and relaxation." In its heyday, Slenderella operated 170 locations in more than fifty cities.

Little by little, however, Bonnie Prudden and a small but growing cadre of fitness enthusiasts began to convince women they could turn to vigorous exercise to hold on to their "honeymoon figure." This promise made exercise palatable for a country obsessed with women's femininity, despite bringing with it tremendous pressures—*there are no ugly women, only lazy ones*, the cosmetics mogul Helena Rubinstein famously quipped.

By the early sixties, Bonnie had become her own brand. She was a spokesperson for Grape-Nuts and Converse sneakers. She released an at-home "gym" with baseball great Mickey Mantle—a kind of isometric resistance band contraption—that featured illustrations of the two stars' faces on the box. (Notably, the box describes the same piece of equipment as Mantle's Minute a Day Gym for men and as Bonnie's Figure Beauty and Vitality Kit for women, promising "A Slimmer, Firmer, Livelier Figure-Up-to-the-Minute Scientifically Balanced Method.") She worked with YMCAs and YWCAs and girls clubs from coast to coast. She hoped to work with the NAACP in the South, writing its leaders that she thought her program could help civil rights workers remain strong and resilient, but the timing never worked out.

When Bonnie's *Sports Illustrated* cover hit newsstands in late summer 1957, she would also introduce Americans to an extension of her brand that would prove as enduring as her fitness philosophies: Exercise could be more fun if you wore special clothing—like a uniform, but with more zest. She had designed her own athleisure wear.

Sports Illustrated's editors had cooked up the cover after Clare Boothe Luce, the wife of Time, Inc., publisher Henry Luce, told her husband that the magazine, launched only a few years earlier in 1954, could be doing more to appeal to women. At Clare Luce's insistence, the publisher hired a group of women consultants to advise on what they wanted to read. The group was led by writer Laura Z. Hobson, author of the novel *Gentleman's Agreement*. It was this crew that suggested showcasing Bonnie.

Inside the magazine, Bonnie's feature offered an enthusiastic sales pitch for exercising for both health and vanity. "You're going to get the results you want," she writes, "a better-looking body, a better-functioning body, but most of all, more energy to enable you to get more fun out of life."

The issue includes a pullout chart for women, advising them to measure every part of themselves weekly. It also asks them to check off their weekly sleep habits, activity, and irritations. (Among the latter, women could choose from "the boss" and "neighbors" to "noise" to "servants"—a reflection of the magazine's well-off audience in its early years.)

The package culminates with a two-page fashion spread, debuting Bonnie's own designs—and the concept of workout wear. Bonnie had always loved clothes, but the options for exercise were limited. Women could buy leotards and tights at specialty dance shops, but such shops could be hard to find. There were cotton gym clothes— baggy T-shirts and shorts cut for men's bodies—but who felt attractive in those? Many women wore blouses with tailored shorts or pants that weren't always comfortable.

Since her days teaching free conditioning classes to children, Bonnie had believed in "outfits" to enhance performance. She required her young students to wear white cotton T-shirts with underwear dyed either canary yellow (for kindergartners) or sky blue (for first and second graders). Older girls wore black long-sleeved leotards. For adults, she advised that exercise clothes be tight, so they could better identify what they wanted to change. "Clothing is the most important thing at the start," she later said. "If you look like a lump and have no pizzazz in yourself, then you are lost."

Bonnie was close friends with the head of the dancewear company Capezio, Ben Sommers, and as early as 1947, she sent him sketches, which he would have "sewn up." Throughout the next two decades, she would work with the company to launch a complete line of fitness fashions—the first real line of exercise wear.

The *Sports Illustrated* spread showcased her line, including her trademark leotite. The outfit, the magazine says, "embodies those qualities one should look for in exercise clothes: ease of movement and a snugness of fit that reveals every bulge on the body." Her leotites, leotards, capri pants, and tops were initially made of cotton and wool blended with DuPont's new miracle fiber, nylon. She sold her fashions through Montgomery Ward, a low-cost retailer with stores across the country. Her signature look would eventually include crop tops—she was proud to show off her unusually firm midriff well into her forties.

Bonnie had stumbled on a kind of magic formula for getting women to listen: fitness *for* femininity. She could have a real impact, it seemed, if she wrapped her fitness advocacy in the trappings of beauty rituals, like broccoli dipped in chocolate.

The formula opened doors in unlikely places.

In the late fifties, she began a pilot program at the Westchester women's prison Westfield State Farm. In a *New York Times* feature on the program, journalist Gay Talese writes of the participants: "They could have been dancers getting in shape for a Watutsi block party. Instead, they were convicted killers, prostitutes, and narcotics addicts exercising to keep fit (and lose weight)." Bonnie had been invited by the prison's superintendent, Talese writes. "Fearful that girls with too much energy might become unruly," the superintendent "regarded Miss Prudden's program as a preventative for riots."

The prison's cafeteria, he noted, was plastered with posters that read:

BE SLIM AND SOPHISTICATED

YOUR SECRET WEAPON: A LOVELY, LISSOME FIGURE

GROUCHY? TIRED? IRRITABLE? COME TO BONNIE PRUDDEN.

For two months, volunteers participated in Bonnie's workouts. At first, "the Westfield girls' muscles ached," Talese wrote. "But they slept soundly. They had larger appetites. They had less nervous tension. Girls who wished to lose weight, lost it. The underweight girls gained. The girls showed signs of grace and poise—even some talent as teachers in this field."

After two months the participants put on an exhibition for the other inmates. They were "grandly applauded," wrote Talese. At the end, ice cream was served.

Not long after her *Sports Illustrated* cover, Bernard "Berney" Geis, a flashy New York City book publisher, saw potential in Bonnie's formula, too, and invited her to codify her figure-shaping methods. While her first three books focused on fitness for the whole family, her fourth went all in on the power of exercise to shape and reduce a woman's body.

Berney Geis had recently founded his own firm, Bernard Geis Associates, thanks to financial backing from some of his top authors, including *House Party* TV host Art Linkletter, comedian Groucho Marx, and Dear Abby's Abigail Van Buren. He was developing a reputation for turning books into sensations—and for shaking up the musty old book publishing industry. As his star publicist, Letty Cottin Pogrebin, who would run four departments by age twenty-two, shared with the writer Brooke Hauser: Until Berney came along, "publishing as a profession spoke in whispers and wore tweed. After Berney, it whooped and hollered." Berney would soon publish Helen Gurley Brown's groundbreaking *Sex and the Single Girl* and a few years later, Jacqueline Susann's *Valley of the Dolls*, a roman à clef about pill-popping starlets. He knew what moved copies.

Berney wanted a book that would capture the most salable part of Bonnie's brand: how exercise could keep you young and make you beautiful. Bonnie knew, after all, that her primary audience was, she later told one reporter, "trapped housewives and mothers who were collecting fat on their hips and thighs."

For a while, the book in progress was called *How to Keep*

Slender and Fit After Forty. But after much discussion, Bonnie agreed to tweak the title to *How to Keep Slender and Fit After Thirty*. Berney explained in a letter, "I haven't spoken to any woman in her late twenties, early thirties or middle thirties who would be particularly eager to buy a book that says 'after forty.' And I haven't spoken to any woman in her forties who admits she would walk into a store and ask for a book that brands her as being over forty."

Besides, in 1961, thirty wasn't the "new twenty." Most women were raising multiple kids by age thirty. Airlines pressured flight attendants to retire by their early thirties. One executive explained, "the average woman's appearance has markedly deteriorated at this age."

For the book, Bonnie teamed up with reporter Dorothy Stull, whom she'd gotten to know through *Sports Illustrated*. "You can't turn back the clock—but you can wind it up again!" promises the back cover copy. In a chapter called "Do You Like What You See in the Mirror?" Bonnie writes: "Go into a room with a large mirror, strip down and take a good look. If what you see pleases you, great. You can be sure of keeping it from now on. If some things look fine, but you'd rather slide over the rest of it—don't. You've been doing just that for some time anyway, and look where it got you." She then adds this bit of encouragement: "As you look over yourself, remember that no matter how bad your shape is, no matter what your age and vitality are, no matter how long you have been in this state, all this can be changed." In one series of photographs, she incorporates a mop into her floor routine. She knew her audience.

At Geis's encouragement, the book also included a chapter on exercises for sex, titled "Sexercise." Its inclusion was almost as scandalous as Helen Gurley Brown's volume, which hit shelves a year after Bonnie's book. "This chapter is not for puritans," Bonnie begins. "If you think that sex is a naughty word, and that any frank discussion of it is shocking, I can only advise you to skip to the next chapter right now." She continues: "My own feelings are quite the opposite. What shocks me is that it is necessary for me to be a pioneer in writing this chapter. As far as I know, this section of the book sets forth in print for the first time the simple, fundamental exercises every normal man and woman should practice in order to enjoy a full, happy and vital sex life. I will never be able to understand why there have not been scores of books published on this subject long ago."

The book became an instant bestseller. The *Atlanta Journal* called it "the most sensible and delightful book on physical fitness ever to be written," and commended Bonnie for doing the "impossible"—making exercise seem like fun. The *Brooklyn Record* called it "wonderful."

When Berney published *Sex and the Single Girl* the following year, Helen Gurley Brown included a chapter titled "The Shape You're In," in which she advises that women, and particularly single women, *must* remain thin and attractive. (Brown herself famously ate almost nothing.) When she discusses taking up exercise, she notes that "a scant handful of women in any one city ever avail themselves of this sure-fire route to sexiness."

She then recommends *How to Keep Slender and Fit After Thirty*, writing, "Miss Prudden is an exerciser from way back, with the figure to prove it. And her book describes about ninety-three hundred thousand things you *could* do if you had a rubber body, and the stamina of King Kong."

No need, she says. Just do a fraction of what she recommends and you, too, can be sexy and gorgeous. "I've been walking up the seven flights to my office just on the strength of this nonsense. And no coronary yet!"

———————————

Slowly, slowly, the country began to come around to exercise. Federal programs encouraged Americans to take walks on their lunch breaks. Offices began to install gyms for their employees. Holly-wood became infatuated with Southern California "beach culture," as a growing roster of films and television series—from Sandra Dee's *Gidget* to Frankie Avalon and Annette Funicello's *Beach Party* movies—showed young, tanned, and increasingly toned beachgoers running around, playing volleyball, and generally having the time of their life.

From the start, however, fitness left huge swaths of the popula-tion behind. "[Exercise] promotion efforts were rarely directed to-ward those who had yet to benefit from the nation's culture of abundance," writes McKenzie. "Exercise was imagined to be a re-placement for the physical activity that had been lost to sedentary, 'desk-bound' work; the nation's lower classes were largely assumed to be engaged in work that had some measure of physicality." Even if they weren't, many poor Americans were denied the leisure time, means, and space to exercise.

For these same reasons, fitness developed a reputation as a white person's pursuit. YMCAs and YWCAs in predominantly Black communities—most Ys were still segregated at mid-century—offered some Black Americans a safe space to move, and Black-owned magazines and newspapers began to advocate for exercise regimens in their lifestyle sections.

As far back as the early twentieth century, exercise offered some Black women a powerful feeling of physical pride that defied soci-ety's relentless message that Black bodies were less valuable than white bodies. "In the early twentieth century, the image of the over-weight, unattractive, and putatively asexual 'mammy' dominated media images," writes historian Ava Purkiss in her study of Black women's fitness. "Physically, the black woman exercise enthusiast was in service to herself whereas the 'mammy' constantly served others," Purkiss continues. "She demonstrated that health, fitness, and beauty did not remain the exclusive domain of white women."

And yet, whatever public and private resources were devoted to helping mid-century America become "fit" were almost exclusively devoted to white communities. It would be decades before this would begin to change.

For middle-class Americans who could afford a television set—and had the time to watch it daily—the small screen led many to adopt an exercise routine for the first time. Television was exploding at the same time as Americans' nascent interest in fitness, and it didn't take long for broadcasters to begin beaming exercise evangelists into living rooms, targeting (who else?) trapped housewives. If the rise of the small screen was partly responsible for the "softening" of the nation, perhaps it could also help reverse the damage.

In these early years of TV, shows were funded entirely by sponsors, and a growing list of food and diet brands lined up to pay for programming. In 1962, an article in the trade magazine *Sponsor* headlined "TV's Great Bust-and-Chest Boom" noted: "Many advertisers are discovering that there's considerable box office appeal in sponsoring programs that convert the female viewer's bulges into alluring curves. And if things continue at the present rate, 'America the Lazy' will soon turn into 'America the Beautiful.'"

For some women, these early fitness programs helped to combat what *The Feminine Mystique* author and feminist icon Betty Friedan had dubbed the "problem with no name"—the malaise and longing for self-determination so many wives and mothers felt—by encouraging them to connect with their bodies and suggesting their happiness mattered. But they could also reinforce it, sending the message that wives owed it to their husbands to be in tip-top physical form—and it was *their* job to ensure their husband and kids stayed fit, too. Fitness was becoming one more item for women to add to their never-ending to-do list.

When NBC's *Home* show invited Bonnie onto the program in 1956, she would become one of first fitness experts to host exercise spots on national television. After NBC canceled *Home*, the network booked her for its fledgling *Today* show, where she convinced host Dave Garroway to roll up his sleeves and sweat along with her on air. (She eventually quit the show when a diet pill company began sponsoring her segment. Viewers assumed she was endorsing the pill, which was neither scientifically sound nor safe; she wanted nothing to do with it.)

In the early sixties, Bonnie got her biggest break yet: television executives offered her her own series, *The Bonnie Prudden Show*, introducing her to an even larger swath of America through syndication.

Bonnie's series, like most other mid-century exercise programs— including the immensely popular *Jack LaLanne Show*, hosted by the charming young strong man of the show's title—aired in the mornings, when many women were cleaning the kitchen or vacuuming the living room for the millionth time and looking for a break. In each short episode, Bonnie would focus on a particular theme— marriage or pregnancy or exercises to do at the office *or even at cocktail parties!* She would demonstrate relevant moves, answer questions from her "mailbag," and interview a special guest.

But like most early women's fitness regimens, Bonnie's show could be a mess of contradictions. An early recording captures these mixed messages to almost absurd effect. The episode features a cheery theme song of women's voices that advise: "Men love you when there's less of you. / Bonnie Prudden lets you see the YOU you really ought to be!" Speaking directly to mothers, Bonnie explains that little boys *and* little girls should exercise. Little boys, she says, need strong bodies to house their brains. Little girls, to develop attractive figures and strong muscles for giving birth. (Oh, and yes, also to build courage.) *No muscle, no curve*, she reminds them.

As the decade progressed, Bonnie's episodes took a more serious tone as she focused on mental health as well as physical health, despite cultural stigma around the subject. She addressed aging parents and alcoholism, depression, and even suicide. She often drew from her own struggles, addressing viewers with her trademark frankness.

The intimacy Bonnie cultivated by talking to women about their bodies created a space to broach other sensitive topics, as she guided viewers in much more than how to limber up or slim down.

————————

Sixty years later, I found myself sitting at Bonnie's mammoth desk—the same desk that once occupied her Madison Avenue–style office in her fitness institute in White Plains, the same desk from which she told reporters America was crumbling. I was surrounded by artifacts of her life: shelves stuffed with magazine and newspaper clippings, closets filled with the leotites she wore in *Sports Illustrated*, walls covered with the art she collected. There was a vast library showcasing the nineteen books she wrote over her lifetime and the work of hundreds of other authors—thinkers, historians, and healers.

In 1992, Bonnie moved to Tucson, Arizona. She gravitated toward the city's warm climate and embrace of holistic medicine. After divorcing Dick Hirschland, she never married again, but instead spent her final thirty-five years living with her close friend and work associate, Enid Whittaker. Bonnie had been *going-going-going* for nearly a century, repeatedly "winding the clock up again," as her books had promised, until time finally stopped for her at age ninety-seven.

It was Enid, a frank and friendly former PE teacher, who had invited me here to immerse myself in Bonnie's life, which she has preserved with extreme care in the modest home they shared. Like much of Bonnie's legacy, her archives have been hidden from public view, tucked away in a living room in the Catalina Foothills, available only to those who seek them out.

As Bonnie moved further into middle age, she began to direct her energy toward a new project: helping people manage pain. In 1976, she developed a system she called Bonnie Prudden Myotherapy. (*Myo* means muscle.) Myotherapy treats aching muscles by applying pressure to trigger points—areas where our muscles have become injured and irritated—and then "reeducating" these muscles with corrective exercises. In her 1980 book, *Pain Erasure*, a *New York Times* bestseller, Bonnie wrote: "This book is designed to help people who hurt or who have friends, relatives or teammates who hurt." Basically everyone. Today, there is a small but devoted community of Myotherapy practitioners around the world—including Enid, who in her mid-eighties continues to treat clients.

During my visit with Enid, as I sat behind Bonnie's desk thumbing through binders of archives, I learned that Bonnie's first home as a married woman was three blocks from my apartment in New York City, on a quiet block on East 74th Street. I thought about the pain Bonnie must have experienced in those walls, in which she had been asked to sacrifice so much of herself to be married, to feel loved—and how movement had helped her manage that pain. If she hadn't cultivated a trust in her body, a physical competence and autonomy rare at the time, she might never have broken free. She might never have become Bonnie Prudden. And I might never have had the opportunity to cultivate a trust in my own body through movement—one that had not only propelled me to (unknowingly) jog past Bonnie's former home countless times while training for road races, but also provided me with the confidence to forge a career, to seek out an equal marriage, to build a life on my own terms.

Back at home in New York, I pulled up a recording of Bonnie's hit *Keep Fit / Be Happy* album on YouTube and felt an invisible cord of connection to the newlywed who, more than eighty years ago, lived up the street. And as I bent and stretched to the dulcet tones of her conditioning cues and the cheerful instrumental soundtrack, I felt the stresses and anxieties particular to my own twenty-first-century life, liberated as it may be, begin to lessen. I felt my shoulders relax. And I realized: Bonnie's work, from the start, was always about finding—and then offering—a refuge from pain. At its best, the fitness movement she launched would do just that.

———————

Back in the early sixties, Bonnie's message was just starting to sink in: Americans could be happier and healthier with regular exercise. And yet for women, this message was confounded by popular culture's equal focus on exercise as a beauty tool—and by the relatively new belief that women's bodies were projects to be molded, improved, and reduced for a lifetime.

Soon London would become the world's cultural epicenter, transforming the way young people around the world thought, dressed, and lived—and fueling the sexual revolution.

More women would grow to appreciate their physical desires and power—and obsess over their figures, which were increasingly on display.

CHAPTER 2

TUCK

What *is* a sexy woman?
Very simple. She is a woman who enjoys sex.

—Helen Gurley Brown, *Sex and the Single Girl*

The world saw so many revolutions in the sixties that the rise of London's skirt hemlines by a few inches may not seem particularly significant. But cultural revolutions often progress in inches, quietly sneaking up until, one day, entire countries look around and find themselves transformed.

While the Beatles and Rolling Stones were lighting up music charts and young women's libidos—and the Pill was allowing women to act on those urges more fearlessly—a young British fashion designer was introducing a new way of thinking about women's clothing that both complemented and accelerated women's simmering desire for liberation. Mary Quant's designs were playful, they were androgynous, and most relevant to the history of women's fitness, they were skimpy. She introduced the world to the miniskirt.

Mary Quant didn't set out to help launch the sexual revolution—or the fitness industry. She didn't explicitly aspire to change the way women viewed their bodies. But as more women bared their skin privately and publicly, more became motivated to refine every contour.

As a design student in the 1950s, Mary Quant was bored with the way Britain's middle- and upper-class women were outfitted. To her eyes, even young people dressed old, with their modest blouses and calf-length skirts, all buttoned up over a flesh-cinching girdle. She wanted to design clothes that were fun. Clothes that complemented her life and her artist friends' lives—lives that included working (outside the home), dating (whoever they wanted), and—as the British music scene revved up—dancing (without parental supervision). Neither Quant's friends nor the teenage baby boomers on their heels wanted to follow their mothers' path to domestic submission. They were optimistic, they wanted to have a good time, and they wanted to look great doing it.

In the mid-1950s, Quant and her husband, Alexander Plunket Greene, opened a boutique called Bazaar on King's Road, a bustling street in Chelsea, the heart of London's burgeoning creative scene.* Quant would become a London it girl, the perfect model for her forward-looking fashion. And the store would help to provide the wardrobe for the Swinging Sixties, fueling what legendary *Vogue* editor Diana Vreeland dubbed in 1965 the decade's "youthquake."

Bazaar sold an eclectic mix of Quant's original designs and accessories made by her art-student friends, and it felt like a party inside. "Drinks for customers enhanced the fun of browsing as duchesses jostled with typists and the thump of jazz spilled out of Bazaar's open door onto the pavement," the writer Juliet Nicolson, who

---

* The space that housed Bazaar is now a Joe & the Juice coffee shop. I'm weeping.

lived on King's Road, wrote in *Harper's Bazaar.* "Passers-by stopped to stare at the eccentric window displays, where models adopted quirky poses, motorbikes serving as props. Suddenly, shopping had become as enfranchised as it was sexy."

In the basement, the couple's friend and business partner, Archie McNair, owned a restaurant that "provided a meeting place for the in-crowd," from the Rolling Stones and rebel Princess Margaret to directors, models, writers, and photographers.

But it was Quant's signature minimalist garment that would start a revolution.

In the 1920s, Americans had been scandalized by flapper dresses, which exposed women's arms, calves, and ankles. Fashion grew increasingly conservative in the decades that followed—but then a new rebellion began. In the late 1950s French haute couture designer André Courrèges featured thigh-grazing skirts in Paris. Quant began experimenting with hemlines soon after, rolling skirts at the waist and trimming them at the bottom. Eventually she gave the style a name—after her favorite car, the Mini Cooper—and brought the look to the masses.

Quant's new miniskirts were simple and colorful. They signaled, as Nicolson put it, "an energetic innocence that belied [their] rebelliousness." They were also affordable, and they sold out almost as soon as they appeared on her clothing racks—joined, in time, by micro-minis and micro-micro-minis. Stores across Britain and then the world began carrying her innovations—which along with minis included waistless dresses, brightly colored tights, PVC raincoats and shoes, hot pants, and waterproof mascara. Designers at other labels soon built on her brand, and her look became the look of the decade.

In many ways, the miniskirt liberated women. It was a lot easier to move in a miniskirt than in the tailored, crinoline-layered skirts their mothers wore; they were short enough to "run, catch a bus, dance," Quant said at the time. Plus, the new, more free-flowing styles didn't require a girdle. But in liberating women from the tyranny of undergarments, the miniskirt also exposed them. Before, women's fashion was designed to flatter the body; now the body had to flatter fashion. Quant knew this. "I didn't get fat even when I was pregnant," she told Britain's *Telegraph* in 2012. "You have to work very hard at staying slim and it's a bore. But it's worth it."

For the many young women who were already captive to the diet culture of the 1950s, the minimalist look gave them one more reason to obsess over their figure. "Until now it was fairly easy to find clothes that helped you hide figure faults," designer Bill Blass commented in *Ladies' Home Journal* in 1965. "But today's pared-down knee-baring fashions have you out in the open now, and the only thing to do is shape up fast." Never mind that, as historian Elizabeth Matelski points out in *Reducing Bodies*, "cotton and textiles are more easily manipulated than flesh and bone."

With more of their limbs exposed, women became increasingly interested in shaping those limbs. Lotte Berk, a German Jewish dancer who fled Nazi persecution for London, would emerge at the exact right moment to give women what they wanted—offering a more sensual flavor of fitness than her American counterparts and giving birth to the global multibillion-dollar barre industry.

———————

Before she became one of Britain's first fitness celebrities, before she made television hosts squirm with her frank talk about a woman's "inner core," Lotte Berk was a dancer without a stage.

While Bonnie Prudden relished her role as America's gym teacher, Lotte thought of herself as an artist, not a "keep fit girl"—a mid-twentieth-century Briticism for women who fancied regular exercise. It was a descriptor she detested. But in pioneering what would become barre, she would build on the nascent idea that in a quest to "keep fit" for fashion, women could reap more meaningful physical rewards, too.

Born Lieselotte Heymansohn in 1913 in Cologne, Germany, Lotte grew up in a wealthy family whose home straddled two streets in the center of the city. Her father owned a successful chain of tailor shops and wanted her to become a concert pianist. But she was always theatrical. "My life was filled with music, but it was not my burning ambition," she once told her grandson. "My body ached to dance." And so, in her late teens, wiry and raven-haired Lotte enrolled at the Mary Wigman Academy of Dance, trailblazers of expressionist movement and modern ballet.

She met her husband, Ernest Berk, who was also a dancer, at the academy; he opened the door when she rang the bell on her first day. Her star soon began to rise in Germany, as she was invited to tour the country and perform solo shows. "I was tasting fame and loving it," she said. In 1934, at twenty-one years old, she gave birth to a daughter, Esther.

But because she was a Jew in Germany amid Hitler's rise to power, everything began to feel precarious. "Fear was like a silent fog that chilled the air," she said of the time. "Soon the air of persecution was seeping into our daily lives." One day, hours before she and Ernest were scheduled to put on a recital, the Gestapo called and warned that if she went onstage, its officers would arrest her. Her husband could perform as planned, since he wasn't Jewish. The police distributed leaflets that read, "If you are a good Nazi you will not attend this performance." In a conversation with her grandson in 1984, she described the night's events this way:

> With my heart thumping I stood hidden backstage in the wings. The director announced that I would not be performing and Ernest would dance as though I was. He gestured for me to come forward. I walked onto the stage and someone

appeared and presented me with a large bouquet of flowers. I retreated clutching the flowers, giving a bow back into the wings as Ernest danced. You could almost see me with him as he gestured to where I would have been had I been dancing. At the end the audience broke into thunderous applause and cried out, 'Dance, Lotte, dance!' I felt triumphant and came forward. More flowers were thrown at my feet. As the applause died down I shouted out to them, 'Thank you for not being Nazis!' Immediately the waiting SS rushed onto the stage screaming, 'Out, out!'

Ernest had inherited a British passport from his grandfather, and this proved to be Lotte's ticket to safety. "Hitler changed my life and Ernest saved it," she later said. In 1938, Lotte, Ernest, and Esther fled to London, where they rented a room in a house crowded with refugees. A few years later, she would learn that her beloved father, who had fled Germany for Holland, had been captured and killed in a gas chamber at Auschwitz. These traumas would shape Lotte's personality in complex ways.

Lotte and Ernest created a bohemian life together in London, surrounded by artists and intellectuals. Britain hadn't yet embraced modern dance, so work was scarce. Ernest bounced between low-paying jobs, and Lotte eked out a living as an art school model, a dance teacher, and a vaudeville-style performer. But not long after arriving in the city—annoyed with Ernest for what she perceived as a lack of ambition—she began an affair with another man. It was the start of a tumultuous open marriage for the couple.

In her 2010 memoir *My Improper Mother and Me*, Lotte's daughter, Esther Fairfax, recounts her mother's love-hate relationship with men. "She had such a natural instinct to flirt, to play the coquette," Fairfax writes. "How quick she was to bed them. How quick she was to throw them out. She was a natural predator with a killer streak." Later, her sexual candor would find its way into her workouts. "Sex came into everything she did," Esther told me. "You know, you *felt* sex from her."

As a mother, Lotte was at turns loving and horrific.* She continually banished Esther to boardinghouses and schools so that she and her latest lover could have free rein of the family apartment. (She would kick out Ernest as well.) When Esther was a teenager, Lotte dared her daughter to perform oral sex on men and convinced her to become a topless dancer in Paris. When the producer of a show in which Lotte and Ernest were performing raped Esther, Lotte told her, "Let's agree to forget about it. We could all lose our jobs."

For most of their adult lives, Lotte would alternately lavish Esther with support or treat her as a fierce rival—one who, in Lotte's eyes, never showed her mother enough gratitude. The two women looked alike and shared similar mannerisms, but Lotte could never forgive Esther for being two decades younger.

In her early forties, Lotte began a romantic relationship with a woman named Cynthia that would set the rest of her life in motion. Cynthia brought out a softer, more joyful side of her. "Cynthia was able to give her the love that no man had managed to," Esther writes in her memoir. Cynthia was also a lifelong drug addict, and her drug of choice during their relationship was morphine. Lotte moved in with Cynthia and fell in love with the opioid, too, injecting herself daily.

When Lotte and Cynthia's relationship ended, Lotte quit the drug, at least temporarily. Heartbroken and in withdrawal, she was restless. "I have got to do something or I am going to go mad," she

---

* Ernest's crimes as a father were also monstrous. In a particularly disturbing incident of sexual assault, he cajoled a twelve-year-old Esther into getting in bed with him naked and pressed his erect penis against her throughout the night. Esther recounts this and many other nightmarish tales of her childhood in her memoir.

told her daughter, pacing around her apartment. "But what can I do?"

Through her circle of artist and intellectual friends, Lotte had grown close with a kind woman (and future Jungian psychologist) named Ann Mankowitz. It was a best friendship that would prove fateful to the future of fitness.

In the 1950s, Ann and her husband, Wolf Mankowitz, suddenly found themselves rubbing elbows with Britain's film stars. Wolf was a successful novelist, playwright, and screenwriter. Later, in 1962, he would play matchmaker around one of the decade's most iconic movie franchises, when he introduced pal and filmmaker Albert "Cubby" Broccoli to Harry Saltzman, who owned the film rights to Ian Fleming's James Bond novels. Broccoli and Saltzman would then coproduce *Dr. No*, the first Bond film, and Wolf would cowrite the screenplay. He would also cowrite the screenplay for the original *Casino Royale*.

After her breakup with Cynthia, Lotte would visit Ann every day, and the two would discuss what Lotte could do with her life. Initially they decided they would open a children's daycare together—until Lotte remembered that she didn't like spending time with kids. (As Esther wrote in her memoir, "the thought of mother looking after little children brought me out in goose pimples.") Ernest encouraged her to do something based on what she knew. She began to consider opening a dance studio not for dancers, but for women who wanted to *look like* dancers.

The idea was novel at the time. Britain, like America, had its sprinkling of gyms and establishments where women could work on correcting their "figure faults," and community centers offered military-style workouts inspired by the Royal Canadian Air Force exercises. But on both sides of the pond, stand-alone studios where women (or men) could attend a group fitness class were basically nonexistent. The world "needed somebody like Lotte to bridge the gap between exercise and dance," Esther told me during an interview. The time was right for something new.

Lotte's workout developed organically. She had injured her back years earlier, and to recover, she devised a series of exercises that combined her modern ballet training with yoga and stretching. The exercises' foundational move was a pelvic tilt, or tuck, in which you roll your groin forward to protect the spine. Lotte had also spent time teaching nonprofessional dancers: Ernest taught amateurs at a local community college, and she occasionally stepped in for him. Her collective experience helped her invent an utterly original and, by the era's standards, rigorous regimen. "It was all instinctual," Esther told me. "It developed, it became, and then it was."

Still, Lotte was reluctant at first. She was an artist—not a teacher, not a "keep fit girl." But she needed something to do. She needed money. And she missed performing.

Then a wealthy friend offered to pay Lotte's first year's rent on a studio if she would "make something of it," and Ann Mankowitz gave her the final push she needed. Ann promised to be her first student—and ask her new celebrity friends to be her classmates.

And so, in 1959, Lotte leased a former women's hat factory to become her studio. It was a dank basement space on Manchester Street, a tucked-away road lined with stately Georgian townhouses in London's chic Marylebone neighborhood. The studio was about a fifteen-minute drive from Mary Quant's Bazaar and just around the corner from EMI Records, the legendary music publishing company that would soon sign the Beatles.

Lotte, then forty-six years old, set to work turning the L-shaped space—which had only one small window, facing another building,

and almost no ventilation—into a workable studio. She installed
green carpet and a tiny loo in the hallway. On one wall, she installed
a ladder of ballet barres from floor to ceiling, for stretching. She installed a single barre around the perimeter of the main classroom.
She named her technique Rehabilitative Exercise. She was ready for
business.

It didn't take long for the green carpet to become Lotte's stage,
every class a performance. She dressed the part, teaching in a leotard
and tights—sometimes fishnets. Her students wore similar dancewear. (Bonnie Prudden's leotites hadn't made their way to London.)

From the start, Lotte attracted fashionable women who were already thin but driven to shape their bodies to perceived perfection.
Ann had made good on her promise and filled the studio with celebrities. That list eventually came to include Bond girl Britt Ekland and
actress Joan Collins. It included journalists and literary stars, among
them the acclaimed Irish novelist Edna O'Brien, who would later
write a prologue to Lotte's first book, *The Lotte Berk Book of Exercises*. ("As a writer," the prologue notes, O'Brien "gets cramped and
stiff, headachy and tense." Lotte's exercises were "the answer to all
these problems.") Barbra Streisand once attended a class, and she allegedly kept her hat on the whole time.

"Go hang yourself," Lotte would tell students as they walked
through the door. "You must always hang before we start. Only then
are you able to warm up."

Students dutifully followed her command. They hooked their
feet into whatever barre matched their height and suspended themselves upside down. Lotte then switched on the record player and
began leading her pupils—often haphazardly, never in quite the
same order—in her exercises. "The classes gave women, maybe for
the first time, a kind of permission to look at themselves," Esther
told me, and to appreciate what their body could do.

As the Swinging Sixties took off, Lotte became a star. Television and radio shows invited her to demonstrate her exercises, and she began popping up in British *Vogue*. Her studio became a place to see and be seen, and her "wicked tongue and sense of humor" helped her build a cult following. Before she hired instructors to work for her, she was teaching seven hours a day, six days a week.

As was true of all of the fitness personalities of the era, Lotte's physique helped her sales pitch. She had always been lithely muscular, thanks to genetics and her training as a dancer. Despite a constant craving for chocolate—she filled her fridge with sweets and little else, except occasionally a sausage—she prioritized staying slim. She began to explicitly promise that her exercises would fail to transform women's bodies only if they were lazy. "Have you ever seen a flabby dancer?" she would ask interviewers. "Of course not. They are firm all over, and that is what I want to offer women." She liked to say that a woman's "muscles should be her corset."

But as much as she reveled in her new lifestyle, Lotte tried to disown her fitness persona, according to her daughter. "With Greta Garbo style, mother would frequently say, 'I don't want to be famous for my exercises. I don't want to be known as a keep fit person. Oh, how I hate those words: *keep fit*. I want to be known for my creative dance, for my artistic talents, to be taken seriously as an Artist,'" Esther writes. "She would raise her eyes to the heavens with arms outstretched in hope that someone would hear her pain."

For former Broadway and George Balanchine dancer Sandi Shapiro, however, Lotte's fitness regimen was a revelation. In 1968, Sandi and her family moved to London, where her husband had accepted a job running the European office of the William Morris talent agency. She missed dancing, but as a young mom, she felt her professional days were behind her. She learned about Lotte's studio through word of mouth. "I remember taking a taxi there and going down the stairs and thinking, *Oh my God. This is horrible. With the dampness and the smelliness and the horrible worn carpet—I'm gonna hate this,*" she told me. "And I didn't."

For the next six years, she attended class four to five times a week. "Part of the reason it felt so exclusive was because it was so different from any other exercise thing that might have been happening in London. The way everything was combined, and how she talked about it—it made it more than what it really was. I mean, if you take each little move apart, it boils down to pretty much nothing. But because of her, it was fantastic."

The more money Lotte made, the more she styled herself to look the part of a Chelsea Girl, complete with a closet full of Mary Quant. She bought herself a Mini Cooper, the car of the era, with *L.B.* painted in gold on each of the doors. "Fame flattered her spirit and the money and success that came with it gave her a lifestyle that she embraced with heart and soul," Esther writes. She even got a Vidal Sassoon bob.

While Mary Quant was revolutionizing how women dressed, the young coiffeur Vidal Sassoon was reinventing how women wore their hair. Sassoon had grown up in poverty, spending seven years of his childhood in an orphanage in London, and he came out of his early life with grit and steely determination. Sassoon's mother had fled pogroms in her home country of Ukraine—she and Vidal's father were both Jewish—and while Vidal was too young to fight in World War II, in his teens he joined an underground group of Jewish veterans dedicated to breaking up fascist meetings in East London. In his twenties, Vidal would apply all of the verve he had cultivated during his young life to his newly discovered passion: hairdressing.

Before Sassoon, stylish middle- and upper-class young white women would, once a week, elaborately style their hair either at home or a beauty salon, coiffing and spraying it into a helmet. Like girdles, these rigid 'dos made it difficult to really *move*. Women carefully avoided messing them up—and many showered only once a week.

Sassoon opened his first salon in London in the mid-fifties and would hone his style throughout the sixties, giving women sleek, low-maintenance cuts that they could more or less wash and wear. He would give Mia Farrow her signature pixie cut for *Rosemary's Baby*, and he would give model turned *Vogue* creative director Grace Coddington her "five-point cut." Sassoon's new approach transformed the way many women began to think about hair, and gradually helped to usher in a new, less fussy era for women's grooming.

It also made it easier for women to exercise. Without having to worry about ruining their carefully crafted bouffant hairdos, women could move their bodies in new ways.

It was natural that Mary Quant and Vidal Sassoon would become friends and collaborators, inspiring each other with their modern minimalist looks. Sassoon cut Quant's hair into one of his iconic bobs, and she designed clothes with his cuts in mind. Quant's models, including supermodel Jean Shrimpton, wore their hair in Sassoon cuts. But like Quant and her miniskirts, Sassoon marketed his haircuts exclusively for a certain kind of woman—an already thin woman.

"I work with the bones of the face," he once told *Weight Watchers* magazine. "If a woman came to me with her bone structure covered by several layers of fat, I would tell her to go home, lose 40 pounds and *then* come back."

From the start, Lotte saw her classes as fuel for the brewing sexual revolution and told friends that she hoped to advance the "state of sex." She talked about her affairs while she taught and playfully disciplined her students with a whip. She named her exercises "the prostitute" and "naughty bottoms." One move was simply called "the sex." Perhaps most famously, she told students, "If you can't tuck, you can't fuck." This kind of frankness in postwar Britain—and everywhere still, really—was radical.

When interviewed, Lotte delighted in asking hosts, "How's your sex life?" and watching them squirm. "When photographed," writes Esther, "she would strike a pose with one hand on her hip, provocatively pushing it to one side."

In the 1970s, British television personality Prue Leith invited Lotte to be a guest on a local women's lifestyle show she hosted.* She had some idea what to expect, since she was also a student. "I went to [her] for weekly torture sessions," Leith writes in her autobiography, *Relish: My Life on a Plate.* "Her language was as strong as her German accent and she was obsessed with the 'inner core,' which included not just abdominal, but also vaginal, muscles."

But any hope that Lotte would tone down her message for polite society was quickly abandoned. "My warnings to Lotte that this was a pre-watershed show proved quite useless," she writes. "She had me lying on my back on the floor while she, seventy if she was a day, tiny, thin as a stick insect, in a black leotard and tights, pranced around like a demented teenager, exhorting us, 'Squeeze, squeeze, make like fucky-fucky. More, more, fucky-fuck, squeeze, squeeze, tighter, tighter. Think of your lover as a string bean: he is getting away, quick, hold on to him, squeeze . . .' I doubt if anyone on the program will ever forget it."

Women came to Lotte to change the way they looked, convinced they needed to mold their bodies to fit a cultural ideal of beauty and unforgiving fashions. But while they tucked, flexed, stretched, and squeezed every muscle in their body, Lotte encouraged them to strengthen their bodies for their own pleasure, too. "Women had

---

* Yes, that Prue of *Great British Baking Show* fame.

unlaced their corsets," Esther told me. "Now they began to unlace and embrace themselves." Lotte's former students describe the classes similarly: They loved how they made them look, but they also appreciated how they made them feel.

It was an enthusiastic Midwesterner—not Lotte herself—who would take barre global.

Lydia Bach didn't initially aspire to fuel a fitness phenomenon. She started her career working as a tax lobbyist for the nonpartisan Taxpayers' Federation of Illinois near her hometown of Decatur. But in the early 1960s, she became disillusioned with government and felt she could do more good traveling the world. Lydia traveled to Syria to do humanitarian work. She traveled to Afghanistan. She taught English in Ethiopia and did aid work in Spain. Eventually, in the late sixties, she followed friends to London.

Lydia arrived as Lotte Berk's fame was peaking. She was never a dancer, but she was athletic growing up, spending her days on the playground jungle gyms and later, in college, joining her boyfriends on ski trips and tennis courts. She'd always liked challenging herself physically. So when her friend Britt Ekland—the Bond girl—told her about an exercise class that offered women a truly challenging workout, she had to check it out. "I was really physically strong," she told me in an interview. "I'd traveled the world by land. So I was shocked when I couldn't do any of the moves."

Lotte hit it off with Lydia right away. Lydia was striking—long and lean with waist-length blond hair and big blue eyes—and charismatic. Both women were direct, adventurous, sensual, and independent. And after a few classes, Lydia was hooked. She loved the way the workout energized her, the way it pushed her physically. "It changed my body," she told me. She became a regular.

One day, seeing her passion for the classes, a friend suggested that she take the workout to New York.

Lydia had been to New York only once, and she hated it.

But she loved a challenge.

She ran the idea by Lotte, who handed over the U.S. and Canadian rights to her technique for several thousand pounds in cash, a percentage of Lydia's future earnings, and the promise of seeing her name go international. Later, according to Esther, Lotte regretted that she parted with these rights so willingly, and without the guidance of a lawyer: When book offers and other business opportunities came her way, she was forced to turn them down, since she no longer owned what she had created.

In the early seventies, New York City was descending into a long period of decay. The Upper East Side, though, remained more or less pristine. The neighborhood had long held a reputation as the most elegant in the city, with its regal brownstones, world-famous museums, and visible wealth. It was home to exactly the kind of woman who might have the time and money to pay someone to help her shape her body.

In April 1971, Lydia opened the Lotte Berk Method studio in a townhouse on 67th Street between Fifth and Madison Avenues. The studio spanned several floors, and instead of green carpet, Lydia went for pink. The larger space—and the bathroom's location inside the studio—made it an instant upgrade from the original. Lydia was renting, and for a while, she was also sleeping on the studio floor.

In the dozen years since Lotte had first started teaching, a handful of other small fitness studios had sprung up in New York and Los Angeles, giving Lydia some competition. Disciples of German strong man Joseph Pilates—the inventor of the eponymous strength and flexibility workout—taught lessons in studios and homes around Manhattan, from an outpost in Henri Bendel's department store to instructors' apartments. *The New York Times* would showcase

Lydia's studio alongside two others, one offering stretching and strengthening from a dance teacher and another acrobatics.

But Lydia had a secret weapon. With Lotte's blessing, she sent out hand-calligraphed invitations to her mentor's New York–based client list—wealthy ladies who had taken classes at Lotte's studio while passing through London—encouraging them to visit her Upper East Side studio. Like its London predecessor, the studio was soon filled with recognizable faces, from Ali MacGraw and Candice Bergen to Princess Lee Radziwill. Later, Lydia told *The New York Observer*, she taught three generations of Kennedys in one class.

In the beginning, the studio remained an exclusively female space. "I felt that women should be able to go someplace and not have to care what they looked like, to be comfortable," Lydia told me. "And I thought, *Fuck you, men, you've got all your clubs around New York City. Now we've got ours.*" But her attitude softened over the decades. She hired a male instructor and began to teach a handful of male students—including the writer Tom Wolfe.

Tom's wife, Sheila, was a client and believer in the workout, and she thought its exercises might help her husband. After years of sitting at desks and writing, the *Bonfire of the Vanities* author was so stiff he could barely reach past his knees. Tom became a client, and six months later, he was able to do a backbend and a split. Tom and Sheila's daughter, the journalist Alexandra Wolfe Schiff, remembers accompanying both her parents to class as a teenager.

"Everybody went there," she told me.

In the beginning, Lydia carried on Lotte's legacy of incorporating sexual frankness into the workout. In that same *New York Times* article about the studio, Lydia described the method as "a combination of modern ballet, yoga, orthopedic exercise and sex." In her 1973 exercise book *Awake! Aware! Alive!*, which features photos of Lydia wearing a sheer leotard, she devotes the entire last chapter to sex. "All of the exercises in this book are important for sex," Lydia advises. (The book's editor at Random House was the legendary Nan Talese, who was also a client at Lydia's studio. Talese told me coyly, "The men in the office used to come and look at the pictures that were spread out on my sofa.") The 1970s American press loved this angle. In a feature that excerpted the book, *Cosmopolitan* gushed in the title, "Exercise Your Way to a Better Sex Life!"

But over time, as American culture shifted, so did the Lotte Berk Method. From the mid-1970s into the 1980s, the idea that women enjoyed sex became less revelatory. Women developed more physical confidence, and Lydia tweaked the method to be more physically rigorous. "I loved the challenge of making it harder, faster, and better," she told me. She hired a growing roster of instructors, mostly former dancers, to teach at the studio and do the same.

By the early 1990s, few of the Lotte Berk Method's American devotees knew anything about its origins. In a 1994 article for *Harper's Bazaar*, journalist Annemarie Iverson wrote of her classmates at the Upper East Side studio: "Most had never met Lotte Berk. Some had no idea that she was a real person who lived in London." One client tells her, "Lotte is the woman with long blond hair." To which Iverson explains, "It was a common mistake: She confused Lotte with Lydia Bach." (The fact that they have the same initials only added to the confusion.) Another client corrects: "No, no, no. There is no single Lotte."

Was she wrong? Lotte did contain multitudes. And before long, the studios teaching her method—or variations thereof—would multiply exponentially. Most would drop references to the workout's creator altogether, partly due to licensing agreements and partly to an evolving clientele, opting instead to align themselves with her exercises' signature piece of equipment: the ballet barre. In the decades that followed, Lydia and her disciples would train nearly all of the women (and one man) who'd go on to open today's biggest barre franchises, from Core Fusion and Physique 57 to Pure Barre and The Bar Method.

————————————

On a steamy Tuesday morning in late July 2019, I traveled an hour and a half west of London to the idyllic country town of Hungerford, Berkshire. Lotte's daughter, Esther Fairfax, lives in a modest home just a short walk from the town's main street, a windy road of shops, pubs, and inns. Esther, then a radiant eighty-five years old, was teaching a 9:30 A.M. class in her home studio—a sun-drenched living room off her kitchen, decorated with abstract oil paintings, light beige carpet, and a white ballet barre around the perimeter.

Today's class, like every class, would be filled with her regulars. One of these regulars, Jennie, had been showing up for forty-seven years.

Dressed in a black leotard, sheer black tights, and a fitted floral shirt, Esther greeted me with a warm smile. She still wears her white hair in a sleek Sassoon-esque bob. She had recently been ill and was relieved to be teaching again after a short hiatus.

"I've really missed this," she told me.

I would be joining her class that morning. I was intrigued to see how contemporary barre had evolved from the original workout— whether, like a game of physical telephone, the technique had been morphed beyond recognition.

Her home was filled with mementos of her life and fitness career—photographs, books, a copy of Lydia Bach's *Awake! Aware! Alive!* Soon students began showing up, a small group of mostly blond British women in their sixties and older, dressed in tank tops and leggings. (Take away their British accents and they could have been my mom's Dance It Off friends at her suburban Atlanta cardio dance studio.)

"All right, let's go!" Esther announced.

We made our way into the living room studio and found our places at the barre, and she switched on a bossa nova CD.

Esther began the class with a gentle warm-up not unlike warm-ups at contemporary barre studios in New York. But as class got going, it was clear that this would not be the serious, intensely choreographed workout I was used to, where the goal of each set of moves, instructors explain, is to work your muscles until they literally quiver. Everyone moved at their own pace and to a slightly different beat. No headset microphone was necessary; we could hear Esther fine without one. And as the class progressed, her students chimed in to remind everyone what exercise came next: "Oh, this one's Sara's favorite." "Bugger, I hate this one." "Time for fold-ups."

I recognized most of the moves, though they did feel something like second cousins to the ones I'd become familiar with in contemporary barre classes. And I was lost in an unfamiliar terminology. Fold-ups—or "fold yourself in half"—were tiny crunches. When Esther told us to make "happy feet," I asked, "You mean, flex?" and she quickly tsk-tsked me: "That sounds too much like the gym." Later, we were instructed to get into what Pure Barre instructors call the pretzel and Esther calls the tramp—a difficult floor position in which one leg is bent in front and the other in back and the hips and butt are rotated forward and lifted. I was the only one in the room who struggled with this one.

About halfway through class, a few students called for Esther to get out the whip, and she revealed a well-worn brown leather weapon. She teasingly tapped me with it during fold-ups, correcting my form with her free hand. Shortly after, during a period of class in which everyone got very quiet, we sat in a circle with our legs crossed and Esther instructed us to "lift, two, three, four, five, and release, two, three, four, five." It took me a moment to realize we were doing Kegels. At some point the music switched from Latin to

French. When we moved on to legwork, Esther told me, "You know, you could be good if you kept coming back."

Class ended and the women walked back into the kitchen, chatty and energized. I was proud I had kept up with them, though my legs felt a little wobbly. (The relaxed vibe was deceiving—I would be sore everywhere for the next two days.) Everyone changed into street clothes around the kitchen table, paid Esther in cash, and said their goodbyes.

When the last student left, Esther turned to me.

"These women have been with me for a long time," she said. "This is my life."

Today, stand-alone barre studios number more than 850 in this country, and that's not counting the one-off classes being taught at gyms like Equinox and other multipurpose studios or the many virtual offerings that emerged during the coronavirus pandemic. Pure Barre's client base alone is more than half a million strong.

While many women still seek out the workout to "lift, tone, burn" their way to a "ballerina body," many stick with it because, as I discovered, it can make you feel good: The first time I returned to barre after giving birth to my son, I left the studio feeling hopeful, proud of myself, and lighter on my feet than I had in months. And when I asked barre-devotee friends and acquaintances why they enjoy the workout, several said it made them feel "energized" or "motivated." Some pointed to its meditative qualities—the workout is so challenging, it requires complete focus, which can be head-clearing. "I forget about what's going on outside the room," my friend Melanie, a forty-year-old human resources director in Connecticut, told me.

Barre is also gentler on the body than workouts that involve a lot of bouncing or pounding. Journalist Samantha Matt wrote in *Women's Health* that barre "totally changed [her] life" by helping her manage her fibromyalgia, a condition that causes full-body pain, stiffness, and fatigue. "When I first felt my muscles tighten after taking a few classes, I immediately became addicted to the burn." And it's widely recommended for pregnant women. It turns out Lotte's obsession with the so-called inner core—the ab muscles and pelvic floor—led to exercises that can help with labor, delivery, and postpartum recovery. My college classmate Sarah, a lawyer living outside Chicago, took barre classes until the day before she gave birth to each of her three children, and she's convinced the workout helped her deliveries go smoothly, telling me: "My ability to push was amazingly impacted."

And then there are the workout's sexual health benefits.

With the Swinging Sixties spirit long extinguished—Lotte Berk's "prostitute" and "sex" moves were long ago renamed—the workout's teeny-tiny resistance movements, performed at a ballet barre, can even make classes feel prim. Instructors rarely draw attention to the fact that the workout can, as many instructors privately admit, bring very real improvements to women's sex lives. "It's kind of like this weird elephant in the room," a barre-going friend in her late twenties who lives in San Francisco told me. "No one talks about it. But after you've done barre for like four days in a row, you're not going to lie there like a dead fish during sex. You feel like a strong woman who's like, *rawwwr*, you know?"

But even without barre being an explicit sex-enhancing workout, women can still reap its benefits—from pelvic floor strength to increased stamina. "I think if we were all pelvic thrusting, holding on to the barre, and the instructor was like, 'This will be so great when you're having sex later!' everyone would immediately get uncomfortable," my San Francisco friend told me.

When Lotte Berk first introduced women to her workout in the sixties, the class's sexual openness felt thrilling and empowering, because it was taboo. Now, more than fifty years after the sexual revolution, turning a rigorous strength-training workout into something overtly sexual feels gratuitous. "I want that hour to myself for my peace and my well-being and my mental health," Burr Leonard, the creator of The Bar Method, told me, echoing the feelings of other women I spoke with. "I think that's what it does most powerfully."

———————————

Back in the early seventies on New York City's Upper East Side, as society ladies and celebrities taxied to class at Lydia Bach's studio, they might have noticed a small cadre of women breaking a sweat right out in the open on Fifth Avenue. Less than two blocks from the barre studio, in and around the city's Central Park, women were discovering the joy of jogging.

CHAPTER 3

Run

If you are losing faith in human nature,
go out and watch a marathon.

—Kathrine Switzer

I t was only a matter of time before women took to the streets for fitness. In the late sixties, as a growing number of American women were demanding equal rights, a small but equally passionate group began fighting for a very specific kind of liberation: the right to run. Their women's movement was about *actual* movement. At the dawn of the seventies, women distance runners likely numbered in the dozens. By the end of the decade, after shedding literal blood, sweat, and tears, they would top tens of thousands—becoming tens of millions today.

The rise of running represented a dramatic shift in the way women viewed their bodies—and their own potential. Running is rarely graceful. (I humbly offer up every race photo I've ever taken as evidence.) It almost always involves breaking a sweat. Before treadmills were widely available, it usually entailed a public display of speed, strength, and self-reliance—or struggle and suffering, depending on the day. It is in no way conventionally feminine.

Bonnie Prudden, Lotte Berk, and a handful of others had introduced middle- and upper-class white women to the benefits of a regular exercise habit and sold the mainstream on exercise as a tool for beauty. Now it would take a kind of athletic superstar to bring women's fitness from the respectable privacy of living rooms and boutique fitness studios onto sidewalks, park paths, and streets—the right woman, at the right time, with the right combination of talent and personality.

Kathrine Switzer, a twenty-year-old journalism and English major at Syracuse University and onetime beauty pageant contestant, was that woman.

Kathrine's mission began on a frigid Wednesday in April 1967, when the college junior, her running coach, and her boyfriend set out in the sleet to run the Boston Marathon. The 26.2-mile course, the oldest marathon in the country, was officially open only to men—authorities believed it was dangerous for a woman to run fast for more than two miles at a time. It was almost as uncommon for grown men to run in those days; most Americans thought of runners as oddballs with a masochistic hobby. A female distance runner was downright concerning. But Kathrine had run thirty-one miles in one stretch while training. She wasn't worried about her health—only about crossing the finish line.

For the first few miles, Kathrine cruised along. She had selected her outfit for the race carefully—looking good made her feel good. That morning, she skillfully applied her makeup; she wore old gray sweats over a maroon tank top and shorts that she dyed special for the occasion, with a plan to toss the sweats once she warmed up. Like the other runners, she had pinned her race number to the front and back of her outer shirt.

When fellow marathoners spotted a woman in their midst—
something that wasn't immediately obvious thanks to her sweats—
most shouted words of encouragement. A few asked for tips to
convince their wives to run. She was feeling buoyant.

Around four miles into the race, a press truck carrying reporters and photographers slowly approached. That's when the trouble
started.

Hey, it's a girl! It's a GIRL! the guys shouted.

"What are you trying to prove?" one yelled.

Nothing! Kathrine thought. *I just want to run.*

It wasn't the first time media had shown an interest in her running. Reporters had shown up when she competed in a men's track
meet a year earlier. She shrugged them off. She was a budding journalist herself. She knew their way.

Then the press guys turned to the race's codirector, John "Jock"
Semple, a cantankerous Scottish American with a notoriously short
fuse, who was riding along with them. They began playfully taunting him: *You let a BROAD in your race, Jock?*

In a matter of seconds Jock snapped—and so did the photographers' cameras.

The race director leapt out of his seat and toward Kathrine. He
was a sight, in his fusty Boston Athletic Association sport coat and
slacks, nostrils flared like a bull's. Before she knew what hit her—
literally—Jock was tackling Kathrine from behind, grabbing at the
number on her sweatshirt and trying to physically remove her from
the course. Kathrine screamed. Her boyfriend, who was training to
be an Olympic hammer thrower, shoved Jock off her and sent him
flying to the curb.

"Run like hell!" Kathrine's coach yelled.

Kathrine was shaken, but she kept going. Now, she knew, no
matter what, she would have to finish the course. But the hits kept
coming. A few minutes later, after fuming about the incident, her

boyfriend, Tom, turned his annoyance on Kathrine. He never wanted her to run the race in the first place, he told her. What *was* she trying to prove? And now, after what he'd done in her defense, he was sure he'd be banned from trying out for the Olympics. *Great.* He abandoned her mid-stride, ripping off his number and running ahead—which she took as a breakup—leaving her in tears. Her emotional pain soon gave way to physical pain when she realized she had developed horrendous blisters that made every step feel like running on glass.

Four hours and twenty minutes after she started the race, Kathrine crossed the finish line. She was exhausted but exhilarated. She believed she had discovered her life's purpose.

I've always admired elite (read: fast) runners, but I used to think of them as being a different species than me. We might love the same sport, but our practice of it looks very different. They are Michelangelo; I'm a fifth grader blithely painting flowers on construction paper. To be sure, running is core to my identity—my sense of self, spirituality, purpose—but my body just wasn't built for speed.

It didn't occur to me until I was researching this book that elite women runners made it possible for me to run my leisurely meditative jogs through city streets and park paths—and to officially enter the New York City Marathon. Nor that, just a few decades ago, women had to fight to do something as fundamentally human as running, which our ancestors did to survive. All women's fitness pioneers have had to break barriers and fight formidable social norms, but those who made it possible for women to run faced hard-and-fast rules, enforced with aggression.

The story of women's running could begin with our prehistoric matriarchs running across savannas. It could begin in Greek mythology, with the story of Atalanta, the royal semi-goddess who outran her power-hungry suitors in a race for her hand in marriage, choosing instead to stay single. It could begin with Melpomene, a nineteenth-century Greek woman who, legend has it, surreptitiously ran in the marathon trials for the first modern Olympics in 1896, when women were banned from participating in the Games. (This beat the original ancient Games, when women were prohibited from *watching* the competition under penalty of death.)

The story of women's running could begin with the athletes who, throughout the first half of the twentieth century, risked social exclusion for participating in the few track events for women that existed; who were told their presence was a distraction to men. Every woman who dared to run in public before the 1970s deserves credit for opening doors for women to move freely and fully; to experience the profound sense of physical autonomy that comes from propelling yourself forward using only your muscle and will. There's a reason our culture has embraced the language of running—*staying the course, going the distance, crossing the finish line*—as metaphors for life and achievement. Running presents a remarkably pure opportunity to challenge oneself—no one else can do it for you. Because of this, the pride running brings can be expansive.

Before the late sixties, athletic officials believed that if a woman ran more than a mile or two at her full capacity, the effort would harm or even kill her. Urban legend held that running would cause a woman to "turn into a man"—grow hair on her face and chest and develop unsightly bulging calves. Others warned it would "turn her into a lesbian." There was also the old chestnut about physical exertion causing a woman's uterus to fall out.

The 1928 Olympics in Amsterdam were partly to blame—they fueled these cultural fears and set women's running back by decades. That summer, for the first time, women could compete in track and field events. Running competitions included (among other events) a 100-meter race and an 800-meter race. The latter—which involves

two laps around a track, or about half a mile—is an especially challenging event. Longer than a sprint, but too short to pace yourself in
any real way, it's a feat for even the toughest competitors. Critics
were convinced the distance would wreck a woman.

The day of the 800-meter race was the hottest of the Games and
suffocatingly humid. But the nine finalists competing—women
from countries around the world, including America and Germany
and Sweden and Japan—had trained, and they were ready. When the
starting gun fired, the women zoomed around the course, pouring
everything they had onto the track before crossing the finish line
and stumbling into the infield.

The problem was, their effort showed. "Every tumble, every gri-
mace the women exhibited during and after the race became evidence," recounted *Runner's World* journalists Rachel Swaby and Kit
Fox. Spectators and media alike were horrified. Reporters covering
the event played it up as a scene of "carnage and weakness"—of
"vomiting and crying, blood pouring out of wounded feet." The *Chicago Tribune* called it "a pitiful spectacle." A reporter for *The New
York Times* later wrote: "The gals dropped in swooning heaps as if
riddled by machine-gun fire."

The message had been received: Any event that encouraged a
woman to punish her "delicate" body to such a degree was a disgrace.
Olympic officials struck the women's 800-meter race from the Games
and wouldn't reinstate it for more than three decades.

The Olympic decision would have ripple effects. High schools
restricted their track programs to boys. Girls who loved to run grew
up with few heroines to emulate. And, as Kathrine Switzer would
discover in 1967, the almighty Amateur Athletic Union, or AAU,
which governed most competitive running events, prohibited women
from participating in races longer than two miles—which were becoming increasingly popular among men.

It didn't help that early twentieth-century educators had come to believe that serious competition of *any* form was bad for girls and women. Instead of encouraging all-out athletics, by the 1930s, women's physical educators promoted curricula devoted to "health, hygiene, posture, games, play, gymnastics, and dance," explains sports historian Jaime Schultz. (Bonnie Prudden had witnessed as much when she visited her daughter's PE class in 1947 and saw the girls playing circle games, a "horrifying" sight that inspired her career in fitness.) Instead of varsity sports, educators introduced intramural "play days," in which young women from different schools would get together for friendly matchups. After the games, participants would mix and mingle over tea or a meal.

Play days allegedly encouraged "an equal opportunity for joyous recreation," argued women's athletics advocate and future first lady Lou Henry Hoover, "instead of overexertion for a few." But by discouraging all girls and women from developing athletic talent, this mindset held everyone back.

By the mid-sixties, however, young women's track clubs were quietly springing up throughout the country. Most were serious groups for serious young athletes, and they would compete against one another in local, regional, and national meets. Still, their coaches grappled with how to help their sport, and their "girls," gain social acceptance—even admiration. Some coaches insisted their runners smile as they cross the finish line, no matter how much pain they were in.

Performing femininity on the track was taken to a new level by Margaret Ellison, a secretary nicknamed Flamin' Mamie for her fiery red hair, who founded the Texas Track Club in 1958 to coach her teen daughter and other local girls. She saw meets as an opportunity to show the world that women runners could be fast *and* feminine. In April 1964, *Sports Illustrated* featured the club on its cover, dubbing the runners Flamin' Mamie's Bouffant Belles—they were the first female track athletes to appear on the front of the magazine.

The three teens pictured *looked* like cover girls, with their big lashes and bigger hair, but they wore a look of determination on their faces as they posed on the track, poised for takeoff.

Inside the magazine, reporter Gilbert Rogin wrote:

The Texas Track Club is celebrated on two counts—its athletic achievements and the uncommon beauty of its girls, who compete in dazzling uniforms, elaborate makeup and majestic hairdos. These hairdos, which are either bouffant or flip if at all possible, may not be aerodynamically sound and may be "out" east of the Hudson, but they are an unqualified sensation at a track meet.

Rogin goes on to reason:

In one sense, the Texas Track Club has done more to promote women's track in the US than if its members had, say, won the national AAU championships. . . . After the age of 10, American girls generally lose interest in running—it is unbecoming and too far out. And American boys generally lose interest in the few girls who take up the sport, the popular belief being that they look like Olive Oyl or Tugboat Annie. The Texas Track Club, however, has shown that you can be beautiful and still run the 100 in 10.9. Because of this delightful anomaly, its members have been a hit.

———————

Throughout the sixties, America gradually began to accept that beauty and athleticism were not, in fact, mutually exclusive. But most people, men and women, still believed a woman's body was far more limited than a man's body, and in such a way that would prevent her from achieving that most arduous feat of endurance and athleticism: running a marathon.

Since the first modern Olympics were held in 1896, the marathon held a vaunted place in the athletic hierarchy. During those inaugural Games, organizers planned a footrace from the town of Marathon, where a great battle between the Greek and Persian armies had taken place in antiquity, to Athens. Legend had it that a general had called on the Greek messenger Pheidippides to travel from Marathon to Athens's Acropolis to alert Athenian leaders that their army had won the battle, and the fastest way to cover the roughly twenty-five miles of treacherous terrain was by foot. Alas, the general had been running the speedy Pheidippides around for days, sending him all over Greece. When he finally arrived in Athens, he announced, "We have won!" Then he fell over and died.

Millennia later, at the first modern Olympics, seventeen men competed in the marathon but only nine finished the race, earning bragging rights for life. Twelve years later, when London hosted the Games, officials arranged for the course to begin at Windsor Castle, where a princess could view the start, and end in a London stadium, where the queen could view the finish—a distance of 26.2 miles. This would become the new marathon standard.

In the early sixties a scattering of women around the world were quietly undertaking marathons on their own, privately discovering the magic of distance running. They ran on beaches and through forest trails, simply because they liked to run. As the decade progressed, a few even snuck into marathon-length road races that had begun popping up in major cities. But because the AAU banned women from officially competing, they were like ghost competitors—authorities did not record their times, nor did they note their participation.

After Kathrine Switzer crossed the finish line of the Boston Marathon in 1967, co-race director Will Cloney told a reporter, "No girls ran in the Boston Marathon. They merely ran on the same course at the same time as the men." (He also told *The New York Times* that if Kathrine had been his daughter, he would "spank her.") But as the press truck's photos of Jock Semple's attempt to thwart Kathrine made their way around the globe, it became harder to deny women entry—to deny that they could, as they say, *go the distance*.

———————

Despite all of these obstacles, one "girl" already *had* gone the distance at Boston—a year before Kathrine Switzer's fateful run. That woman was Roberta "Bobbi" Gibb. Her story had inspired Kathrine to enter the race in the first place.

In 1966 Bobbi had crashed the marathon, finishing the course in an impressive three hours, twenty-one minutes, and forty seconds. Then twenty-three years old, she was a newly married art student who had grown up in the Boston suburb of Winchester. She had fallen in love with the race two years earlier when her father took her to cheer on its runners, and she became singularly focused on running it.

For nearly two years, Bobbi trained daily, wearing a black one-piece bathing suit, Bermuda shorts, and leather nurse's shoes. She ran in the woods near her family's home and along the Massachusetts coast. When she took a cross-country road trip, she ran across the plains and up the mountains of the West. At one point, she decided to try and cover a hundred-mile equestrian race in New Hampshire on foot and ran sixty miles in two days.

Long, lean, and blond, Bobbi didn't care much about appearance—or most of the other things women seemed to care about in her town. She didn't wear jewelry or makeup. She felt a powerful connection to the earth, and she would sleep outside under the stars, even in the rain. When she ran, she was often accompanied by a pack of neighborhood dogs. She loved to paint murals on sheds and ponder the meaning of life and existence.

When she was a little girl, Bobbi's father, an engineer, had instilled in her a deep appreciation for and curiosity about the natural world. But as she grew up, he and her conventional (or, in Bobbi's mind, *repressed*) mother expected her to settle down, marry, have children, and forget whatever personal ambitions she might have.

Her parents did not approve of their daughter sleeping outside, nor did they approve of her running. They became concerned about what they perceived as her difficulty "adjusting" to adult life. They scheduled an appointment with a psychiatrist.

His only diagnosis was that her priorities were different from those of other young women.

Shortly before the 1966 Boston Marathon, Bobbi had given in and married a friend with whom she hoped she could forge an equal partnership. Her parents were relieved. Then, the evening before the race, she told them about her plans to run, and they again rang up the doctor.

A few months earlier, Bobbi had written the Boston Athletic Association to ask for an application. They wrote her back, explaining that, *sorry*, the race was open only to men. They were simply following the guidelines established by the Amateur Athletic Union, which stated that it was dangerous for women to compete in races longer than two miles. She was furious and heartbroken.

She decided she would run it anyway. What had started as an act of love became something bigger. She was tired of other people telling her what her limitations were. She was tired of people questioning her passions. She was tired of being told she had the mind to be a physicist, "if only" she hadn't been a woman. The race became not only a personal goal but a protest: If she could show the world that a woman could run a *marathon*, perhaps they would reevaluate other so-called truths about what women could and couldn't do. Perhaps she could show other women what they could do, too.

The morning of the race, she slipped a baggy gray hoodie over her black bathing suit and wore her younger brother's shorts, which needed to be cinched with a piece of string to keep from falling down. As runners gathered near the starting line, she hung low and hid behind a nearby row of bushes. To pull off her goal, she reasoned, she would have to first make it to the start without anyone noticing.

When the gun fired, she joined the crowd of runners and almost blended in. But they soon spotted her—a woman! *Are you going to go all the way?* they asked excitedly. She politely told them that was her plan.

She was a curiosity among the runners and cheering sections along the course, but because she was running "unofficially"—without a number—she managed to complete the race and cross the finish line without getting tackled. Or maybe she just had the good fortune of not catching Jock Semple's attention. At the finish line, the governor of Massachusetts, John Volpe, shook her hand. She had run the course faster than two-thirds of the competitors.

The next morning, she was featured on the front page of Boston's *Record American* tabloid, with the headline "Hub Bride First Gal to Run Marathon." From there, her story spread. In May 1966, *Sports Illustrated* covered her feat, noting, "Boston was unprepared for the shapely blonde housewife who came out of the bushes to crush male egos and steal the show." The impact, however, remained to be seen.

Kathrine Switzer had heard about Bobbi from a friend and was awed. She knew it would be significant for another woman to run Boston, but when she scanned the race's rule book, she was surprised to find that it didn't say anything about women entering one way or another. Nor did the application ask runners to indicate their gender. Still, when she applied, she used her first initials, making her K. V. Switzer. She had taken to using K. V. Switzer as her journalism by-line in student papers, inspired by her literary idol, J. D. Salinger.

She was officially accepted into the race.

Kathrine and her coach at Syracuse University, a mailman named Arnie Briggs, trained together, until they finally covered 26.2 miles in practice. But Kathrine didn't want to have any doubts that she could cover the course, so she pushed them to run an additional five miles. At the end, Arnie collapsed into her arms.

The morning of the race, Kathrine fueled up with a huge breakfast of bacon, eggs, pancakes, toast, juice, coffee—the works. The race didn't start till noon, so she would have time to digest. She was nervous and excited at the same time and prayed that she would have the courage to finish if things got tough.

Then the starting gun blasted, and they were off.

The main difference between Kathrine's and Bobbi Gibb's runs was pinned to the front and back of Kathrine's sweatshirt: her official race bib—number 261. It was this bib that would incense Jock Semple. It was one thing for a woman to crash his cherished race as a kind of stunt. It was another for her to masquerade as an official competitor.

Also unlike Bobbi, Kathrine wasn't explicitly running to make a point—to "prove" anything to anyone but herself, and maybe Arnie and Tom. But as the shock of Jock's attack sunk in, her thinking shifted. How dare someone tell her she couldn't run.

It's hard to stay angry while you're running—endorphins have a similar effect on the brain as antidepressants. Over the marathon course, Kathrine's rage turned to motivation. When this was all over, she told herself, she would work to change things. She would show Jock and all the other men like him.

As Kathrine crossed the finish line, no one arrested her, but no governor stood waiting to shake her hand, either. A few days later, her team learned that they had been banned from the Amateur Athletic Union for violating the rules. But as photos of Jock Semple's attack made their way around the world, plastered across newspapers and magazines, a growing chorus began to hail her as a hero.

Soon *The Tonight Show* with Johnny Carson invited her onto the program. At first Johnny playfully teased Kathrine, who wore a stylish bob and a flouncy dress for the occasion. "I'm sure Carson and his staff were hoping for a funny show," she wrote in her 2007 memoir, *Marathon Woman: Running the Race to Revolutionize Women's Sports*. "But when I was on the air, I didn't want to castigate anyone as a fuddy-duddy or make light of the marathon race."

She continued: "Carson could tell I was serious and changed the tone to one of informed support. He had been a track athlete himself, I could tell he understood, and that was great."

———————————

What became the women's liberation movement coalesced around many issues, but they could all be boiled down to feminist leader Betty Friedan's *Good Housekeeping* headline of nearly a decade earlier that preceded her hugely influential *The Feminine Mystique*: "Women Are People, Too!" Feminists fighting social norms and sexist laws wanted men and women to be treated as equals. They wanted women to have control over their bodies, to be able to choose how to use (or not use) them. *The personal is political*, they explained.

What symbolized women's power and self-sufficiency more than actual muscle? The early seventies would see a groundswell of cultural and even political support for women athletes, which would fuel the rise of women's fitness in both direct and indirect ways.

There was the mega-bestselling 1968 book *Aerobics*, by an Oklahoma-born physician and former U.S. Air Force officer named Dr. Kenneth H. Cooper. Before *Aerobics*, few had heard the titular word, which comes from the Greek words for air and life. The book was based on Cooper's work with airmen and astronauts, through whom he discovered that by strategically stressing the cardiovascular and pulmonary systems with exercise, one could improve overall health. It sold millions of copies—and crucially, provided scientifically backed evidence that women could benefit in the exact same way as men from vigorous exercise.

In 1972, President Richard Nixon took the monumental step of signing into federal law Title IX, which declared that all educational institutions receiving federal funding had to provide equal opportunities to men and women. Suddenly, schools' athletic budgets could not be funneled solely into men's sports. Girls thus had more opportunities to play—and receive scholarships—and their participation in sports soared.

The following year, tennis phenom Billie Jean King would beat retired champion Bobby Riggs in a match billed as the "Battle of the Sexes," after Riggs boasted that even the best women's player in the world couldn't beat a man. Fifty million Americans tuned in to watch the two compete in the Houston Astrodome, and Billie Jean King's win was celebrated as a triumph for all women.

It also got some people thinking. Maybe women *weren't* weaker than men. Maybe men just had more opportunities to cultivate muscle. Maybe they were treated as stronger since birth—and when you're told you're stronger, you believe it. With Billie Jean and more women athletes being hailed as heroes, women were encouraged like never before to consider their physical potential.

In many ways, the women's movement and women's fitness promoters appeared to be at odds. Neither Betty Friedan nor Gloria Steinem would dream of publicly endorsing the claims in women's magazines that a woman needed to look a certain way to please a man; that women should exercise because "men love you when there's less of you." In 1965, Helen Gurley Brown had taken over and reinvented *Cosmopolitan* magazine following the stratospheric success of *Sex and the Single Girl*, believing that she was empowering women by sharing secrets for beauty and sex appeal; many feminists laughed at this premise. In 1972, Steinem co-founded *Ms.* magazine to offer an alternative to the hugely influential women's glossies, to explicitly encourage women to be strong and independent.

But social change is rarely tidy; it is human. And the still-new field of women's fitness straddled the old and the new, the patriarchal and the feminist, in complex ways.

While it was easy for feminists to get behind women's sports, which were plainly about opportunity and strength, women's fitness culture posed more of a challenge—even though, as more and more women discovered, regardless of one's initial motivation for starting a fitness regimen, regular exercise could change a woman's entire view of herself and her life. It could cultivate inner strength as well as physical muscle.

In 1971, with its groundbreaking book *Our Bodies, Ourselves*, the feminist Boston Women's Health Book Collective wanted to empower women to better understand their bodies so they wouldn't have to rely solely on the expertise of (mostly male) doctors. In a section titled "Women in Motion," the authors stress the importance of exercise for mental and physical health, before methodically breaking down all of the social and economic forces that prevented women from exercising until that point. They list jogging first in their list of recommended physical activities.

But was there anything *wrong* with wanting to like what you saw in the mirror? Was it possible for a woman to wear makeup and formfitting clothes to please *herself*, or had she just been brainwashed by the patriarchy? Gloria Steinem herself had risen to fame in part because she was conventionally beautiful and slim and feminine and glamorous. There was also Letty Cottin Pogrebin. In the years after working as a wunderkind book publicist for Bonnie

Prudden's *How to Keep Slender and Fit After Thirty* and *Sex and the Single Girl*, Pogrebin had written a bestselling women's empowerment tome titled *How to Make It in a Man's World* and teamed up with Steinem to become a founding editor of *Ms.* magazine. She was also slim and conventionally beautiful.

Running offered a kind of bridge. It was both a serious sport *and* a form of recreational exercise—one in which women were proving themselves to be as capable as men *and* one billed as improving your figure. Feminists could advocate for it with a clear conscience, and women with no interest in feminism could take it up without feeling especially transgressive.

Kathrine Switzer was an ideal front woman for the cause. Like Gloria Steinem, she projected strength and independence. Also like Steinem, she was conventionally attractive enough, slender enough, feminine enough, to get mainstream America to listen. Kathrine liked looking good, and she chose her race outfits with special care. She ran with a girlish ribbon tying up her thick brown hair, pre-race lipstick applied, and nails painted. She was in many ways a white middle-class Everywoman—with star power.

In the early seventies, women's movement leaders hoped to recruit Kathrine to be an official voice for the cause, but she didn't think of herself as political. Some feminists encouraged her to blame the patriarchy, full stop, for inequalities in women's running—as embodied by Jock Semple—but she demurred. Sure, most of the Amateur Athletic Union officials banning women from competition were men. But men had also encouraged her, trained her, given her opportunities from the start. She instead directed all her energy to changing what she could in her own world.

After the Boston Marathon, Kathrine had almost immediately begun working to create more opportunities for women distance runners. If Boston wouldn't let women officially run, *fine*—she would organize her own co-ed races. Over the next few years,

enlightened male race directors from around the world began inviting her to compete in their events as a kind of celebrity participant.

Women runners were slowly beginning to show up at events.
With every passing year, a few more women also began "unofficially" running the Boston Marathon—and running it fast. As
women's athletics became a political issue in the lead-up to the passage of Title IX, women's demands for inclusion grew from a few
passionate voices to a roar.

Finally, in 1972, two months before the passage of Title IX,
women runners scored their first big win: Boston Marathon co-
directors Jock Semple and Will Cloney announced that women could
officially enter the race—as long as they could run it in three hours
and thirty minutes.

"And so, uh . . . you ladies are welcome at Boston," Jock announced at a welcome party. "But you have to meet the men's qualifying time!"

Kathrine had continued to train since her first Boston Marathon,
and she had shaved off more than an hour from her original time.
She qualified easily. Not that she would have missed the event.

As women runners wearing official numbers gathered at the
start line that year, Kathrine could feel the moment's historic significance.* "We were free to be athletes and no longer had to run
carrying the banner of the whole female sex," she would later write.
"Fifty years earlier, people had been afraid to let women exercise

---

* She also felt Jock Semple grab her—again. "I let out a little cry, thinking for a
moment that he was going to hit me," she wrote in her memoir. "But instead he
flashed a big grin and turned me toward the cameras with his arm around me and
said, 'C'mon, lass, let's get a wee bit o' notoriety.' And then he planted a big kiss
on my cheek." Kathrine, generous of spirit as she was, accepted the gesture as an
apology. She and Jock would go on to forge a friendship that lasted until his death
in 1988.

their brains. Until 1972, people were afraid to let women exercise their bodies." Kathrine's work, however, was just beginning.

New York City was becoming a hub for the nation's burgeoning running scene. Central Park's rolling hills and picturesque reservoir made for ideal training routes, despite the fact that the park was becoming increasingly crime-ridden. Taking to the park's paths or city sidewalks after being crammed into an elevator or cubicle or subway car all day felt uniquely freeing.

But the main reason New York became a running hub was a charismatic Romanian garment industry worker who dreamt big. Fred Lebow, raised Orthodox Jewish, grew up in Transylvania and emigrated to New York City after World War II. He attended the Fashion Institute of Technology in the 1960s and began manufacturing fashionable knockoff apparel in the years after. But his true love was running.

New York City's local running club, the New York Road Runners, was founded in 1958 by the Black distance-running pioneer Ted Corbitt and had grown from about 40 members in the late 1950s to 250 members by the end of the 1960s. Fred Lebow had gotten increasingly involved in the club throughout the decade, both as a runner and an organizer, and in 1970, he spearheaded the very first New York City Marathon—which boasted 127 entrants, 55 finishers, and a $1 entry fee. (The inaugural marathon included a singular woman runner, Nina Kuscsik, who had to drop out mid-race due to illness; she later returned to win the women's division.) By 1972, Fred became the Road Runners' president. Inspired by the popularity of the marathon, he had a vision: crowds of runners filling city streets in big-deal races funded by sponsors.

A few years earlier, Fred had met Kathrine Switzer at a road race in New York, and the two hit it off. Kathrine shared some of the same starry-eyed dreams as Fred. She, too, had begun to fantasize about organizing big races—races that would welcome women. A few weeks after that history-making 1972 Boston Marathon, Fred called Kathrine in Syracuse and asked if she might help him with an exciting event he was planning.

The company S. C. Johnson was introducing a new product—a women's shaving gel called Crazylegs. It wanted to capitalize on the hype around women's running, and it figured: What better way to do this than with an all-women marathon? The company hoped Fred would be up for organizing such an event in New York City.

It would be the first ever all-women's road race.

There was just one problem—only a few known women marathoners lived in the city. Fred worried he would be able to enlist only a handful of participants; the optics wouldn't be great. Instead, he proposed a six-mile race, or one loop around Central Park. With fashion always on his mind, he suggested they call it a mini-marathon—named, of course, for Mary Quant's miniskirt.

S. C. Johnson loved it.

With just over six weeks to pull the whole thing together, Fred hoped Kathrine, along with New York City Marathon pioneer Nina Kuscsik, would be interested in organizing it with him. Kathrine was thrilled. Another opportunity to make history!

After six weeks of furious planning, Kathrine drove down to New York City. Days before the race, together with Nina and Fred, the three went on a grassroots publicity blitz throughout the city to convince as many women as possible to register. They hit a popular nightclub north of Union Square called Max's Kansas City—a haunt of glam rockers and pop artists, from Patti Smith to Andy Warhol—where they approached women with cocktails and cigarettes in hand. They handed out race flyers on street corners.

Their blitz worked. In the end, seventy-eight women signed up to run the inaugural Crazylegs Mini-Marathon—a huge number at the time. Race morning was buzzing with women in matching T-shirts with *Crazylegs* printed on the front. Most wore short shorts for ease of movement, resulting in a sea of smooth bare legs, which made the sponsor happy. In a final flourish and a move that feminists could debate for eternity, Fred recruited Playboy Bunnies to appear at the starting line and pose for pictures.

The race was a smash, and it got Kathrine thinking: Maybe women-only road races were the secret to helping women distance runners gain even greater acceptance. After all, in a race with only women, no runner's time would have to be qualified: She finished first—*among the women*. Women could shine on their own. Plus, she liked the image of crowds of women running in public.

Their Boston victory was significant, but Kathrine and other women runners had already begun to set their sights on a bigger goal: an Olympic marathon. Until the Games allowed women to cover the same distance as men, they argued, girls around the world would grow up believing women's bodies were limited. Their dreams would have a hard stop.

―――――――――

As baby boomers came of age in the seventies, many found running to be more than a form of exercise. They found in it something deep—something *far out*. Some ran to connect with the earth and nature. Some ran in quest of a higher level of consciousness, comparing the "runner's high"—a feeling of well-being or euphoria many experience when endorphins are released—to the high of doing mind-altering drugs. Others ran for the feeling of self-control it gave them, in a world where everything seemed to be shifting around them.

The more popular it got, the more running found critics, too. As runners took to streets in droves, many non-runners lamented having to share the road—and would sometimes drive runners *off* the road in frustration. Runners claimed those behind the wheel were just jealous of their glowing good health, and they developed a reputation for having a superiority complex—for believing they were *morally* better than their sedentary neighbors.

The decade saw the creation of running-specific magazines, including *Runner's World*, and a slew of running guidebooks. *The Complete Book of Running*, published in 1977 by a journalist named Jim Fixx, would become a sensation—the defining manual on the subject. Fixx had been a 220-pound chain-smoker who spent most of his days bent over a desk writing and editing magazine copy, until running transformed his body and his life. He became a household name and, for years, the face of the sport. His story ended tragically when, in 1984, at fifty-two years old, he suffered a heart attack and died after going for his daily run. His death would rattle runners everywhere, but he had already made converts out of millions of Americans.

Running slowly began to influence pop culture, too. Celebrities took up the workout, infusing it with glamour. The July 4, 1977, issue of *People* magazine featured *Charlie's Angels* megastar Farrah Fawcett-Majors and her husband, *Six Million Dollar Man* star Lee Majors, on its cover. The couple is pictured mid-jog, feathered manes blowing in the wind, with the headline "Farrah & Lee & Everyone's Doing It: Stars Join the Jogging Craze." Farrah wore a tight T-shirt with *Ferrari* emblazoned on the front, and Lee wore a jacket unzipped to his belly button, revealing his tanned, hairy chest.

Inside the magazine, celebrities from Shirley MacLaine to Tom Brokaw gushed about how jogging had changed their lives. "Jogging once was humbly billed as the common man's most salutary of cheap thrills, standard equipment being a pair of sneakers and the inclination to run oneself silly in the cause of fitness," the article begins. "Kiss those days goodbye. Acting from a variety of more complicated motives—vanity, sanity, even higher consciousness—media stars of every stripe are now falling for the jogging craze, steadfastly bobbing down the toniest streets of Manhattan, Washington and Beverly Hills—risking hit-and-runs, muggings and shin splints for the oddly catching pleasure."

In a few years, Americans would be humming Bob Seger's "Against the Wind," a hit inspired by the artist's days running cross-country. They would draw inspiration from *Chariots of Fire*, the 1981 film about British track stars training for the 1924 Olympics, which nabbed the Oscar for Best Picture.

Women's entry into running was a trickle at first, then a deluge. While men launched the running movement, women would turn it into a cultural phenomenon. Women-specific running books began crowding shelves in the late seventies and early eighties, from *Sports Illustrated Running for Women* to manuals with titles like *Running for Health and Beauty* and *The Beauty of Running*. These books addressed everything from hairdos to husbands to the inevitable catcalls and other harassment (or worse) women might face on the streets.

Many were inspired to run by imagining how it would transform their appearance—this was almost universally sold as its most enticing benefit for women. Some saw how much their brothers or boyfriends or husbands enjoyed running and wanted to try it for themselves. Others wanted a healthy habit to "balance out" the fact that they smoked, or a new activity to keep their minds off smoking when they quit.

But while the promise of physical transformation or health might have gotten them to slip on sneakers, growing numbers stuck with it when they discovered more profound benefits. Hitting the road was freedom—from the drudgery of housework, from martyring themselves for others, from being told they couldn't.

In the fall of 1977, the power of women's running was put on full display for the nation. That November, leaders of the women's movement—Bella Abzug, Gloria Steinem, and others—were planning a national conference at Sam Houston Coliseum in Houston, Texas. The tagline for the conference was "American Women on the Move," and to kick it off, the event would begin with a 2,600-mile torch relay from Seneca Falls, New York—where the women's suffrage movement was launched in 1848—to Houston. Runners would also carry a scroll bearing the movement's Declaration of Sentiments, written by commissioner and poet Maya Angelou. At the end of the relay, female Olympians would hand the torch and scroll to three first ladies of the United States.

Conference leaders asked Kathrine Switzer to start the relay, and this time, she happily accepted.

On September 28, President Carter's daughter-in-law "unfurled a great hand-lettered scroll" and read the movement's Declaration of Sentiments in a candlelit ceremony. Early the next morning, "I ran quietly through the dawn mists of Seneca Falls," Kathrine recalled, carrying the majestic torch.

For the next several weeks, women runners passed the flame from one to another, revealing their physical joy and strength to a rapt nation. The relay went smoothly until the torch crossed the Mason-Dixon Line. In his book *Reaganland*, the historian Rick Perlstein writes:

> Truckers tried to run torchbearers off the side of the road. The Birmingham Road Runners Club, recruited to supply participants, canceled after a pressure campaign. . . . A panicked phone call produced a nineteen-year-old marathoner from Houston who saved the day by covering sixteen miles along the most symbolically powerful leg—the stretch of Highway 80 where Martin Luther King Jr. and his pilgrims had marched to Montgomery for voting rights in 1965. A woman in the tiny town of Prattville watched her pass: "Now why would a woman want to get involved in

something like that for? There's no law against it. But it takes her femininity away."

In the last mile of the relay, the torch was carried by three women: a Black runner, a Latina runner, and the teen who had heroically joined the relay in Alabama. "Hundreds fell in behind them," writes Perlstein, "Bella Abzug leading the way in hat and high heels."

The runners arrived at the stadium to massive cheers.

Running offered a beautiful metaphor for liberation, but even a cursory glance at mainstream pop culture's depiction of runners, and of who was actually hitting the streets, was revealing. Running evangelists claimed the sport was for everyone—*all you need is a comfortable pair of shoes!* But throughout the seventies, the sport developed a reputation for being a favorite pastime of the white middle and upper classes: Having the leisure time to run, having the money to pay for race fees, and feeling safe enough to run outside were largely privileges of these communities. Americans of color risked their safety every time they hit the streets in sneakers.

In the late sixties and early seventies, some Black organizations, including YMCAs in predominantly Black communities, did promote jogging, writes historian Shelly McKenzie in *Getting Physical*. "African American newspapers reported on the new exercise, the establishment of local jogging clubs, and the development of trails and parks, but to a lesser degree than other publications." The founder of the New York Road Runners, Ted Corbitt, was himself Black. But throughout the 1970s, only a slim percentage of Black Americans participated in the activity.

America had a celebrated tradition of elite Black track and field champions. In 1936, sprinter and long jumper Jesse Owens was credited with "single-handedly crushing Hitler's myth of Aryan supremacy" when he won four gold medals at the Berlin Olympics—and yet President Franklin D. Roosevelt failed to invite him to the White House to shake his hand after his feat. In 1960, sprinter Wilma Rudolph became the first American woman to win three gold medals at a single Olympics. But while many cheered the country's Black runners in competition, outside of the professional and Olympic arenas, those who wanted to run for fun or fitness endured harassment and worse. "In the early years, most joggers were forced to contend with taunts from drivers, but Black runners faced particularly harsh conditions," writes McKenzie. "The racist assumption that an African American jogger might be fleeing, possibly from a crime, has long plagued Black men."

Black women were doubly vulnerable.

When the Black distance running pioneer Marilyn Bevans trained in Baltimore in the sixties and seventies, she dodged beer cans hurled at her and, once, a firecracker. She ran with a transistor radio, which helped to tune out racist taunts. Even when Bevans triumphed on the racecourse—she became the first Black woman to run a sub-three-hour marathon—she wasn't always celebrated. "When some runners ran, there were cheers. When I ran, you heard crickets. I was called the N-word sometimes," she told *Runner's World* in 2013. "But I have a slow reaction time. If you curse me out now, tomorrow I would get mad. That was a blessing."

Black distance runners faced racism among fellow joggers, too. "White runners occasionally expressed surprise at the sight of Black runners, based on a racist stereotype that African Americans were incapable of running long distances and were only capable sprinters," writes McKenzie. "This view, which applied to both leisure and sports running, derived from the belief that victory in longer races depended on strategy and training. Short-distance runners, in contrast, were said to win because of sheer physical ability."

Despite the damning obstacles Black runners faced, magazines intended for Black audiences increasingly featured jogging stories and tips, recommending the activity to combat the sedentary life. In the second half of the decade, *Ebony* and *Jet* highlighted Black celebrities and notables from Eartha Kitt and Cicely Tyson to Newark mayor Kenneth Gibson who jogged as part of a healthy lifestyle. In 1980, *Essence* even called running its "favorite" aerobic exercise and sang its benefits.

But relatively few Black Americans felt comfortable enough to make themselves publicly vulnerable in the way that running outside requires, denying Black communities the many physical and emotional benefits the activity offered so many white Americans.

———————————

As more women took up running, more began dreaming up ways to improve their runs. While women entrepreneurs were still rare in the seventies—until the passage of the Equal Credit Opportunity Act in 1974, women business owners couldn't even apply for their own line of credit without a man's permission—running would launch some of the decade's most successful businesswomen.

The biggest commercial breakthrough for women's running— and arguably, women's fitness in general—was launched in 1977 by a twenty-eight-year-old artist in Burlington, Vermont, who would invent a game-changing undergarment.

Lisa Z. Lindahl started running in the mid-seventies when she found herself putting on weight for the first time. She worked as a low-level filing clerk during the day, which meant a lot of sitting, and she sold stained-glass windows at craft fairs on weekends. When a friend raved about how much he loved running, she decided to give it a try.

Lisa had epilepsy, and doctors didn't think it was safe for her to drive—or do much of anything on her own. Her condition made her feel dependent on her husband, Al, a seminary student whom she had married in her early twenties. "At the time, my lack of mobility felt a greater disability to me than having the occasional epileptic seizure," she later wrote. Running offered her an unprecedented feeling of freedom. "By the time I was running an average of 30 miles a week, my body—that same body that had routinely, unexpectedly, violently betrayed me with every frightening and painful epileptic convulsion—had become a strong, reliable friend," she wrote. The only problem was it made her boobs hurt. There was no such thing yet as a sports bra.

Like many full-breasted women at the time, Lisa would sometimes run in a bra that was a size too small to attempt to keep her boobs in place. She heard that other runners would wear two bras to try to create compression. Women with small breasts often ran bra-less. (On her *People* cover, Farrah Fawcett-Majors appears to be among this contingent.)

One morning, Lisa and her sister, Victoria, commiserated over the phone about their breast woes. Then the sisters half joked: Why not invent a kind of jockstrap for women's breasts?

The more Lisa thought about it, the better the idea seemed. She felt compelled to act on it.

Her best friend since junior high school, Polly Smith, happened to be a seamstress, and she was living in Burlington for the summer working as a costume designer for a summer Shakespeare festival. Lisa asked Polly if she could help.

At first Polly demurred—bras were notoriously difficult to design, given the engineering they entailed. But Lisa persisted, and eventually Polly agreed to give it a go. She began to work on the bra at the theater, after hours. Polly's assistant for the summer, a student named Hinda Miller who loved to ski and had recently started jogging herself, was intrigued. She offered up her help, and the three joined forces.

After several failed attempts—Polly would sew a prototype; Lisa and Hinda would run in it and report back on its shortcomings—they got a bolt of inspiration. During a work session in Lisa's house, Lisa's husband Al wanted to give the women a laugh. Six-four with a red beard, he emerged at the top of their staircase bare-chested—or bare-chested except for an *actual* jockstrap he had pulled over his head, "causing the pouch to stretch over his chest in a *most* bra-like way." While strutting down to the living room, he announced, "Ladies! Ladies! Your work is done! . . . I present your jock bra!"

After chuckling, the women wondered: *Wait—could they work with this?*

Polly got to work sewing two jockstraps together. Lisa and Hinda took her prototype for test runs. *Bingo!* The bra was comfortable *and* supportive. "Designers of bras had always been men, so whatever they fantasized about boobs was what happened," Hinda told me in an interview. "We said, 'Form follows function.'"

The women considered officially naming their invention the Jock Bra. But they learned that calling a woman a jock was still pejorative in the South. Instead, they christened it the Jogbra and launched the Burlington-based company of the same name. Shortly afterward, Polly moved back to New York City, where she would go on to work as a costume designer for Jim Henson and the Muppets. But Lisa and Hinda were fully committed to Jogbra. After initially enlisting local women to hand-sew the bras, they eventually began working with a South Carolina factory to produce them in large quantities.

Bringing their product to market presented a seemingly endless series of challenges.* They had introduced their bra through mail-order ads in the back of women's and running magazines, inviting readers to purchase directly from the company. (An early ad read:

---

* To help navigate these challenges, Lisa joined a local group of Burlington entrepreneurs, which also included Ben Cohen and Jerry Greenfield, of Ben & Jerry's ice cream. So the next time someone asks you what the sports bra, Kermit the Frog, and Ben & Jerry's have in common—now you know.

JOGBRA. NO MAN-MADE SPORTING BRA CAN TOUCH IT.) Demand was greater than they could have dreamed, which meant scrambling to figure out how to produce and ship enough product.

When their business model required them to begin selling their bras through retail, they knew that as a small start-up, they had little hope of getting sold in big department stores. Instead, they approached sporting goods shops, many of whose owners balked at carrying "lingerie" alongside footballs and fishing rods. But the women were savvy: They packaged the bras in sporty plastic bags that could be hung neatly on shelves. And instead of adhering to traditional cup and chest sizes, for ease of production and economy of shelf space, their bras came in only three options: small, medium, and large.

By the time Jogbra sold to Playtex Apparel in 1990, the sports bra was an icon of women's fitness and liberation. The original prototypes are now enshrined in the Smithsonian's National Museum of American History in Washington.

With so many women running, how could the Olympic committee *not* introduce a women's marathon? It seemed obvious enough, but proponents would have to prove not only that there were enough world-class women marathoners from at least twenty-five countries on two continents to compete in such an event, but that doing so was not dangerous. Fifty years after the 1928 Olympics in Amsterdam, in spite of all the progress, some still believed it would result in another "pitiful spectacle."

The more women took up running, the less America worried about the dangers it posed to women's health. But fitness as a field of study was still new, and little research existed yet. In Germany, a physician and coach named Dr. Ernst van Aaken had been arguing that because women have a higher percentage of body fat than men and evolved to endure the grueling demands of childbirth, they were actually *better* equipped than men to run long distances. His work inspired others, who were chipping away at dated and sexist beliefs.

Most people were fairly convinced at this point that running would not cause a woman's uterus to fall out, as once feared, but other concerns involving uteri persisted—specifically, about exercise's impact on a woman's period. A University of Minnesota graduate student in American studies and mother of three young kids would soon become inspired to investigate.

Judy Lutter's entry into running was not planned. Her husband, Hap, was a surgical resident at the university, and he ran for twenty minutes every night to relieve stress. One evening in 1973, when Hap returned from his nightly jog, Judy, then thirty-three years old, told her family on a whim, *Okay—my turn.*

She jogged out the front door of their home in shoes she'd purchased at Woolworth's and started down the road. When she glanced back, she saw her kids' faces pressed against a window. She was in as much shock as they were.

She ran for about a mile and was delighted by how energized she felt. Running soon became her nightly ritual, too. Having never played sports—she was a bookworm growing up, and her only physical activity came from Girl Scout camping trips—she was surprised to discover she was fast. Her mile eventually grew to 26.2 miles, and by the mid-seventies, she was running among top competitors at Boston and other marathons.

Whenever she'd place in a race, newspapers would print her name—and the fact that, by then, she was a researcher at the university, completing coursework for a doctorate in American studies. She began to get calls from other women runners who respected her athletic and professional stature—intimate calls asking whether running had disrupted her menstrual cycle, as it seemed to be affecting theirs.

Judy hadn't noticed any changes, but she figured it would be easy enough to find answers. She was surprised to discover basically nothing. She could find little contemporary research on exercise and periods, nor on exercise and everyday women's reproductive health generally.

What she did find was antiquated hearsay, driven mostly by fear. Until the seventies, most doctors believed girls and women shouldn't exercise during their periods—their fragile constitutions couldn't handle it. And practically speaking, for a long time, women had a hard time partaking in vigorous activities while menstruating even if they wanted to. Although the first tampons became commercially available in 1936, for many years, wearing them was controversial. It wasn't until the 1960s that they went mainstream. Their rise was both fueled by and helped to fuel women's growing interest in fitness, as ads relentlessly pitched tampons for "the active woman." (Tampon companies went so hard on the active pitch that Tampax released an ad in the late sixties promoting the fact that its products were also for women who *didn't* enjoy being active—whose favorite activities included shopping, sunbathing, and getting driven around in cabs: "Even if your favorite sports are the spectator variety, there are lots of reasons for using Tampax tampons.")

By the late seventies, tampon ads had shamelessly co-opted the language of women's liberation: Tampons, the ads claimed, were about liberation, plain and simple. *"Feel free!"* one 1978 Tampax campaign proclaimed. "Why let your period slow you down? . . . Swim! Sun! Enjoy! Nothing gets in your way. Be as active as you want to be every day."

Women had the gear—they just needed the information.

Judy decided to remedy the situation. She and a friend created a survey that asked women runners a list of questions about their participation in the sport and everything from periods to pregnancy to menopause. They handed it out at local races and gathered more than two hundred responses. Inspired, in 1978, they got permission to distribute a longer survey at that year's Boston Marathon, and they received 422 responses by mail, many of which included lengthy notes from runners about their personal experiences.

Their responses were illuminating and would provide the foundation for future studies. Judy and a small team gradually began to reveal the benefits of running and other vigorous exercise to women's sexual health and overall health.

After conducting research for several years, in 1982, Judy launched the Melpomene Institute, a nonprofit named for the fabled woman who allegedly snuck into the marathon trials for the first modern Olympics. It was the first organization fully dedicated to researching the effects of physical activity on women's and girls' bodies and lives.

In time, the institute's researchers were joined by a growing number of experts working to show the world that distance running did not pose a danger to women. Collectively, their research would provide essential fuel for the Olympic cause.

Kathrine Switzer wondered: What would make it *impossible* for Olympic officials to say no? She knew women's running had gone global, but how could she prove it? She thought about New York's Crazylegs Mini-Marathon, which had continued to expand, and which had opened her eyes to the ways women-only races could showcase women's speed *and* interest in the sport.

Kathrine had moved from Syracuse to New York City, where she eventually took a day job doing communications and marketing at an athletic equipment company. She had continued to train, too, believing that, in order to be taken seriously as an activist and athlete, she would have to get *good*. In 1974, she won the women's division of the New York City Marathon, and the following year, she came in second at Boston, where she finished in an astounding two hours and fifty-one minutes. She also continued to work with Fred Lebow and the New York Road Runners. She had helped Fred broker a deal for Greek shipping magnate Aristotle Onassis's Olympic Airways to sponsor the New York City Marathon, which brought glamour—and big bucks—to the event. She also volunteered to do publicity for races, which led to TV appearances on NBC's *Today* show and other national programs. If anyone could make an Olympic marathon happen, she could.

After thinking over the situation, Kathrine had an idea: Why not organize a women's marathon series that would take place *all over the world*? Not only would this show Olympic officials that the sport was popular in at least twenty-five countries, but it would reveal the champion caliber of women runners, too. Kathrine suspected such a series would unearth talent the running community didn't even know existed by offering many women their first chance to compete.

First, though, she would need a sponsor. Throughout the seventies, executives had begun to realize they could capitalize on feminism to hawk whatever they were selling. Virginia Slims cigarette ads told women, "You've come a long way, baby!" Tampax had leaned into women's empowerment with its "Feel Free!" campaign. Nike launched a women's shoe called the Liberator. A few years later, one of its ads declared: "Put an end to women's suffrage." (Get it?)

Smaller companies wanted in, too. After Crazylegs had to pull out as a sponsor of New York's Mini-Marathon—the NFL player Elroy "Crazylegs" Hirsch sued the brand for appropriating his nickname—the cosmetics company Bonne Bell stepped in to take its place, followed by the pantyhose maker L'eggs. Surely others would be interested in the exposure of a global women's race series. That's when Avon came calling.

As the world's largest direct-sales cosmetics company, Avon boasted a million representatives around the world. And its executives wanted to invest in women's sports.

At first Avon wanted to focus on women's tennis. It would be sponsoring a training league for Billie Jean King's women-only circuit. But it had started to dabble in running, too. At a luncheon organized by the newly formed Women's Sports Foundation, Avon's executive vice president, Mark Williams, introduced himself to Kathrine. Would she consider advising the company on a marathon it was planning with its Atlanta office?

Kathrine decided to do one better. Over a weekend, she wrote up her dream proposal for an international series of Avon-sponsored women's road races.

Avon helped women feel beautiful, Kathrine figured—just like running. She'd grown up with the brand, her neighbors selling it door to door. Her mom bought "bags and bags of Somewhere Cream Sachet, Honeysuckle cologne, compacts, and lipsticks." The more Kathrine thought about it, the more Avon seemed the *perfect* sponsor. Like running, the "heart and soul of it was participatory, and success came from individual effort—the more you put into it, the more you got out of it."

Kathrine put every race fantasy she'd ever had into her proposal. Even the most well-organized road races were still bare-bones affairs in those days, often without bathrooms or water stations along the course (both of which are fixtures today). Kathrine envisioned "feminine touches, such as flowers everywhere, the T-shirt being a fashion item, clean toilets with tampons, real jewelry (instead of ugly trophies) as commemorative awards and a festive atmosphere."

Avon went for it.

In 1977 the company hired Kathrine full time, and later that year, she launched the Avon International Running Circuit. The series kicked off with the Avon International Marathon in Atlanta. More than 150 runners from eight countries participated, including fourteen of the twenty-four fastest women in the world. Winners received gold and silver necklaces with a charm of Atalanta, the royal running goddess. Every runner got not only a stylish Avon T-shirt but also a cosmetic—often lipstick or powder—in their goodie bag.

Momentum was building. In 1979, Nike, already a multimillion-dollar shoe company, adopted the cause. It placed ads in running magazines, declaring: *We think it's time the IOC stopped running away from women runners*. The ads encouraged readers to send the company letters of support, which it would present to Olympic officials. Nike also created its International Runners Committee, which would lobby for the cause.

Still, the Olympic committee dragged its feet. When an official vote took place in 1980, delegates opted "to postpone the decision on [a] women's marathon until the necessary data and experience are available," according to the committee's minutes, citing a need for "more medicoscientific research studies and experience."

A global outcry erupted, and the committee agreed to vote again the following year.

This time, Kathrine and the many other women's running activists triumphed. In 1981, the International Olympic Committee announced: The 1984 Olympic Games in Los Angeles would feature the first-ever Olympic women's marathon.

———

The Olympics would be taking place in Ronald Reagan's adopted hometown, and the president pulled out all the stops. As the Cold War with the Soviets raged on, Reagan saw the Games as an opportunity to show the world how wonderful—how abundant—life in a democracy could be. The Opening Ceremony, held in the Los Angeles Memorial Coliseum, was a spectacle, paying homage to America's pioneer spirit and pop culture. At one point, eighty-five grand pianos appeared to play George Gershwin's classic "Rhapsody in Blue."

ABC News had hired Kathrine Switzer to provide live television commentary during the marathon. On August 5, 1984, she put on a sharp blue blazer and arrived at the network's Los Angeles studio. She took a moment to revel in the moment. Olympic Marathon Day was finally here. Then she got to work.

With millions of people tuning in to watch the race and more than 90,000 live spectators, runners would start on the track of Santa Monica College and run through Venice and Culver City before entering Los Angeles. They would finish at the Memorial Coliseum.

American Joan Benoit, a twenty-seven-year-old from Freeport, Maine, pulled ahead of the other runners almost immediately and maintained a sizable lead for the entire race. When Benoit strode into the coliseum, she took off and waved her white painter's hat, and the crowd exploded. She crossed the finish line in 2:24:52—a time that would have beat the 1952 Olympic men's marathon champion and all the fastest men's times before that. She then took a victory lap to roaring crowds. Kathrine counted it as her own.

For millions of American women watching the 1984 Olympics, the marathon was revelatory. In the decades that followed, the number of women runners would grow exponentially. The sport hit another milestone in 1994, when Oprah Winfrey ran a marathon and told fans: If I can do it, *anyone* can do it.

Today, more than half of American marathon participants are women. In 2016, at age thirty-five, I joined their ranks as one of the 18,638 women who finished the New York City Marathon that year. I was not fast—a cabdriver once asked me my time, and when I told him, he responded, "So . . . you walked?"—but for me, speed wasn't the point. Deciding and training to run 26.2 miles through the streets of New York City—and then doing it, alongside my then-sixty-eight-year-old dad—brought me as much joy, pride, confidence as anything I have ever accomplished.

The first Olympic marathon inspired untold numbers of women. And yet millions more would identify with one of the opening ceremony acts of the Games. During that lavish spectacle, as a massive orchestra played "America the Beautiful," dancers from around the country formed a map of the United States on the field. Among them were a contingent of smiling ladies in leotards.

They were the women of Jazzercise.

CHAPTER 4

Bounce

Just think—not a single employer, employee,
spouse or offspring in sight. Just you and people
in the same shoes you're in, dancing up a storm.

—Jazzercise print advertisement, 1985

Freedom means different things to different women. In the late
seventies, while thousands were lacing up jogging shoes, others were slipping into a leotard for the first time since girlhood—and
slipping out of the house to dance to Donna Summer's "Hot Stuff"
until their spandex was soaked with sweat.

Freedom, for them, was aerobic dancing.

When U.S. Air Force physician Dr. Ken Cooper coined the word
aerobics to describe his system of conditioning pilots and astronauts,
he never in his wildest fantasies imagined that the term would come
to define a pulsing, neon-hued, mostly female subculture.

But in the years after Cooper convinced more Americans to

make exercise a regular part of their lives, women discovered that dancing—when done regularly, vigorously, *aerobically*—made them feel happy. It made them feel strong. Americans of a certain age had grown up believing that for exercise to count, it had to feel like work—regardless of how many times Bonnie Prudden told them *keeping fit can be fun!*

Dancing? That was something you did at a party. Dancing was pleasure and play.

This belief lured waves of women who had never exercised before through the doors of studios and community centers to try aerobic dancing—which involved at least thirty minutes of vigorous movement to music—for the first time. Dancing felt safe, particularly for women uninterested in smashing any gender barriers. Dancing was conventionally feminine; dance classes were a popular activity for little girls. Few men felt threatened by a room full of mostly middle-class moms shimmying to Tina Turner.

And yet aerobic dancing—eventually shortened to simply *aerobics*—would transform women's lives. It would offer a respite from work and caring for their families. It would create thousands of jobs and first-time business owners, allowing women to support themselves financially. It would offer an opportunity to participate in a group physical activity outside the limited arenas of high school and college sports. And it would introduce many to the joy and power of feeling in control and proud of their own bodies for the first time. By the early 1990s, nearly 30 million American women participated in aerobics, making it the country's most popular fitness activity after walking.

My mom discovered aerobics in the early 1980s, when I was a toddler. She had never exercised in any formal way until then. But when Jan, a neighbor friend, mentioned she was checking out a dance exercise class at a nearby shopping mall in our Atlanta suburb, my mom was intrigued. Her days as a stay-at-home mom to me and my older sister could be monotonous and exhausting, and by the time my dad, a physician, got home from work, she needed a break.

My mom accompanied Jan to class, and she was hooked. She loved the music, the energy, the adult company; she also began to look forward to the endorphin high. She and my dad had met at a disco in the late seventies, and now that she was again dressed in Lycra and losing herself in the beat, aerobics didn't feel that far off from her former nightlife, minus the cigarettes and vodka.

My mom recently shared that one of her most vivid memories from this time involves aerobics: One particularly long day, she had been counting down the hours until class. Finally, in the late afternoon, she changed into her leotard, tights, sweatband, and sneakers. Then my dad called to check in and remind her he had a meeting that night. She had completely forgotten. Deflated, she sat down at the kitchen table and started to cry. Taking in the ridiculous combination of her aerobics costume and tears only made her cry harder.

(My mom's aerobics studio eventually offered babysitting, and one of my earliest memories is sitting in the back of her light gray Buick as she drove to class, then playing in the kids' corner to the sound of muffled instructor cues and Whitney Houston riffs.)

On a scale grander than barre or even running, the rise of aerobic dancing in the seventies and early eighties changed the rhythm of women's days. It changed how they dressed. It changed how they saw themselves and how others saw them. Aerobics had become such a part of the cultural fabric that when the 1984 Los Angeles Olympics committee planned the Games' opening events, meant to showcase the most iconic of American popular institutions, they invited Jazzercise creator Judi Sheppard Missett—a lanky dancer from Iowa with permed blond hair and a megawatt smile—to run in the torch relay and featured three hundred of her instructors in the opening ceremony.

But like the fitness movements that came before it, this cultural domination didn't just spring into being overnight. Aerobics first had to be invented and sold in a way that made women feel like it was something they couldn't live without.

In 1969, Judi Sheppard Missett began teaching adult dance classes for fun and fitness, ushering in a new chapter in exercise, and feminist, history.

Here's what women of the early eighties would have seen when they pressed play on a 1983 home workout video called *Let's Jazzercise*. Against a white backdrop, there is Judi Sheppard Missett, her head high atop her long neck, her bronzed body impossibly limber in a shiny yellow Lycra leotard. As the warm-up gets going, she gives cues with an excitement that borders on mania—*We're gonna get JAZZY, sugar!*—her Midwestern timbre cracking mid-sentence. She is all exaggerated smiles and pizzazz, channeled into moves that seem designed to take up as much space as possible, her long arms and legs expanding and contracting to the beat. Later in the workout she wears a jaunty white bow tie as she dances to "Boogie Woogie Bugle Boy." She is peculiar, she is over-the-top, she is extra. She is the physical embodiment of jazz hands.

She is putting on a show.

When the cameras stopped rolling, a shyer Judi would emerge. The real Judi was earnest and passionate, yes—when we spoke by phone, she peppered our conversations with liberal doses of *gosh!*—but deeply private and reserved. The daughter of a father who worked for the U.S. Army Corps of Engineers and a mother who worked as an accountant, she was a savvy businesswoman with a formidable work ethic. By the time *Let's Jazzercise* was released, Judi was also a self-made multimillionaire, helming and serving as the face of one of the country's fastest-growing franchises. But when she first came up with the idea to teach jazz-dance-inspired exercises to non-dancers, it was her special alchemy of smarts, showmanship, and humility—presented in a lithe, blond-haired, blue-eyed package—that inspired middle-class women to start sweating.

Born in 1944, Judith "Judy" Sheppard grew up in the small Iowa farming town of Red Oak. (She changed her name from Judy to Judi with an *i* before her freshman year of college to seem sexier and more sophisticated.) When Judi was just a toddler, a dance instructor had spotted her moving to a beat while out and about one day and told her mother, *That baby's got talent!* Her mom took the cue and promptly enrolled her daughter in dance classes.

As she grew up, Judi became a star in Red Oak (population: 5,276) and then across the Midwest, wowing farmers at county fairs with routines that showcased her extraordinary flexibility. She could contort her body into jaw-dropping positions, drawing gasps and standing ovations from audiences. One signature move, in which she would bend over backward, grab her ankles, and walk across a stage, earned her the nickname Upside-Down Girl.

In 1962, Judi took off for Northwestern University, where she majored in speech while launching a professional dance career. She'd set her sights on the school when she discovered it shared a hometown with the esteemed Gus Giordano Jazz Dance Chicago—the first studio in America dedicated exclusively to jazz dance (her favorite), run by its "godfather."

Like Judi, Gus Giordano was from the Midwest—he grew up in St. Louis. He began his career performing in shows for U.S. troops during World War II before moving to New York City to dance in Broadway productions including *Paint Your Wagon* and *On the Town*. But Gus quickly discovered he was more excited about choreographing and spreading the gospel of jazz dance than performing. In 1953, he and his wife, Peg, moved to Chicago and opened his three-story studio in the suburb of Evanston.

Gus believed that, unlike more traditional forms of dance, jazz "emanates from the soul, the emotional and physical core of our being." His performances were sleek and fluid and sexy. "Gus's style was challenging, precise, and full of pent-up passion," Judi later recalled in her 2019 book, *Building a Business with a Beat: Leadership Lessons from Jazzercise—An Empire Built on Passion, Purpose, and Heart*. For a farm girl who had never had a serious boyfriend, this was thrilling. She nabbed a spot in his dance company and worked with the master to polish her technique. With dreams of a career in show business, she also booked modeling jobs and auto show appearances and dinner theater gigs throughout Chicago. She performed in "industrial theater" productions—a *Mad Men*–era tradition in which big companies presented their products to distributors in the form of song-and-dance routines—landing gigs with American stalwarts like Westinghouse Electric and U.S. Steel.

Judi's romantic life began to flourish, too. Her junior year of college, a friend set her up on a blind date with a journalism major from Virginia, named Jack Missett. Jack was a modern kind of guy, and he appreciated Judi's thoroughly modern ambition. They clicked. "He said that what attracted him to me was my independence," she later wrote. "I didn't play dumb," and "I didn't hide that I had dreams, ideas, and goals of my own."

In 1966, with Judi fresh out of college and Jack completing his senior year, the couple married. Two years later, they had their first child, a daughter they named Shanna. Judi continued to land gigs—she had even managed to hide her pregnancy from the manager of a nightclub where she regularly performed—but as she took on the demands of motherhood, she began to yearn for more stability in her work. She loved to dance, but her hours were erratic and her paychecks unreliable, and she didn't want to rely on Jack for income. "By age 25, I was living my number one dream," she wrote. "But financial independence? My number two dream was still just that."

Judi began to mull over the idea of teaching. She had taught her first dance class when she was just thirteen years old, when a group of little girls in Red Oak asked for lessons. She even managed to grow the classes into a pint-size business, earning money for college. Teaching wasn't glamorous, but she came alive in front of a class. Teaching, after all, was a kind of performance.

In the summer of 1969, Gus asked Judi if she would be interested in leading a new Saturday-morning class called Jazz Dance for Adult Beginners. Most of the women who had signed up were moms of girls already taking classes at the studio. "They were there anyway—knitting, reading, sitting around waiting for their kids," she wrote. "Why not dance a little themselves?"

Judi agreed. She carefully selected music and choreographed simple jazz routines.

At first her students were excited to learn. But after a few weeks, she saw a depressing *90 percent* dropout rate. *What had she done wrong?* She sincerely wanted to find out, so she began calling her dropouts and asking for answers.

The class, they told her, just wasn't fun. It was too hard. It was demoralizing. "I hated seeing all the things I *couldn't* do in the mirror," one woman told her. "I'll never be on Broadway," another said. "I just want to look good for my high school reunion this fall." She heard the same refrain over and over: The women didn't want to be professional dancers, they just wanted to *look* like them.

It was the same thing Lotte Berk's disciples had wanted—but unlike Lotte's students, Judi's acolytes were not socialites and models and Bond girls looking to tone their bodies to perfection through gentle torture. They were regular Midwestern moms. They wanted to drop a few pounds, and they wanted to enjoy themselves during their precious time away from work and home.

As Judi thought about their responses, a lightbulb went off.

Why not teach a dance class for regular women focused less on technique and more on sweat? A class that approached dance not as art per se, but as exercise and fun?

Judi ran her idea by Gus. He gave her the go-ahead, "so long as it occurred downstairs in the rarely used back studio." She posted flyers advertising a new adult class called Jazz Dance for Fun and Fitness. And she personally appealed to her dropouts to come back and give her another chance.

On the first day of class, instead of standing in the front of the room, Judi positioned herself at the back—turning the fifteen women who showed up away from the mirror. For music, she chose Top 40 hits by popular groups like Creedence Clearwater Revival and Neil Diamond. There was no choreography—she told her students to simply follow her lead as she led them through very basic steps. *Let me be your mirror,* she said. Once the class started, she shouted a constant stream of *Looking good, ladies!*

Gus had instilled in her a belief that every dance performance should be an "emotional journey" with a beginning, middle, and end. She applied the same concept to her class, opening with a warm-up, building to an aerobic peak, then cooling down. After the last song ended, the room broke out in spontaneous applause, "for me and for themselves," Judi wrote. "Without the mirror, they'd engaged the theater of their minds, seeing themselves as active participants in a theatrical performance, rather than passive, non-dancing audience members."

Within a few weeks, her class had grown to sixty students—the most the room could hold. She added more classes to accommodate the interest.

Not all of the other professional jazz dancers at the studio understood or appreciated the classes' popularity. Some accused Judi of "bastardizing" their art form. But when she began to hear her students refer to the classes as "their time," she knew she had created something special.

Jazzercise had been born.

––––––––––––

Before she started teaching adult women, Judi Sheppard Missett hadn't spent much time thinking about fitness per se. She had one of Bonnie Prudden's *Keep Fit / Be Happy* records lying around somewhere. But while she was new to the nascent fitness industry, her program, she would later learn, was building on a centuries-old tradition of exercising to music and reinventing it for the modern woman.

Since ancient times, humans around the world have recognized the power of music to move not only the body but also the soul, incorporating it into both sacred and social rituals. European fitness pioneers in the eighteenth and nineteenth centuries attempted to harness this power to encourage exercise, specifically, by teaching their "gymnastics" programs to up-tempo beats. One nineteenth-century fitness enthusiast observed, "I believe five times as much muscle can be coaxed out, under this delightful stimulus, as without it."

Musicologists call this impulse to move *groove*. We now know the brain is "hardwired to hear music as an invitation to move," writes Kelly McGonigal, a Stanford University psychologist and longtime cardio dance instructor, in her book *The Joy of Movement: How Exercise Helps Us Find Happiness, Hope, Connection, and Courage.* "For most people, the impulse to synchronize our bodies to a beat is so strong, it takes effort to suppress it." Neuroscientists have discovered that music in fact activates the brain's "motor loop"—the regions that plan, coordinate, and time movement. "The stronger the musical beat or the more you like what you hear, the more feverishly these regions consume fuel," writes McGonigal. "It's as if your brain can't hear music without recruiting the rest of the body."

The first American to create a formal exercise program set to music was an educator named Catharine Beecher, sister of abolitionist and author Harriet Beecher Stowe. Catharine Beecher believed that, thanks to industrialization, American women no longer boasted the "superior health and activity" of earlier generations, but had become "feeble, sickly, and ugly."

She studied European fitness programs, and in 1821 opened a private school for girls in Hartford, Connecticut, where she began teaching her workout. The program involved calisthenics that were "exhilarating and amusing . . . graceful movements performed in time to rhythmic music (usually played on a piano)." She even instructed the girls to hold "hand weights" made from oblong cotton bags filled with corn. Over time, she wrote books detailing her regimen and proselytized about its benefits in lectures, influencing school-based fitness for decades to come.

The fitness pioneers of mid-twentieth-century America recognized the power of music, too. Through the "bed ballets" she performed while recovering from her broken pelvis, Bonnie Prudden had concluded music was key to making exercise fun. In the sixties, inspired by innovators like Prudden, YMCAs began to offer their own versions of figure-shaping calisthenics set to music. Lotte Berk brought rock and roll to exercise, teaching her tucks to the Beatles.

They were all onto something. But it wasn't until the seventies that Americans began to see the potential in dance, specifically, as a formal path to improved health for adults.

———————

The seventies were becoming a decade *defined* by dance. The era saw the rise of discos, which offered a respite from the nation's social and political turmoil and whose lifeblood was the pulsing, euphoric music that kept clubgoers on the dance floor until the wee hours. (That, and cocaine.) Americans did the Hustle, the Bus Stop, the Bump, and the Roller Coaster until they could no longer stand. In 1977, *Saturday Night Fever* would pay homage to America's disco kings and queens and catapult John Travolta to stardom. Made for just $3.5 million, the film brought in more than $237 million worldwide. Its soundtrack, which was mostly written and performed by the Bee Gees, was the bestselling soundtrack of all time until 1992, when it was surpassed by Whitney Houston's *The Bodyguard*.

Then there was the smash Broadway hit *A Chorus Line*, which riveted audiences with its tale of professional dancers' triumphs and heartbreaks. The show won the Pulitzer Prize for Drama and the Tony Award for Best Musical and inspired nonprofessionals to want to move.

America's obsession with dance fueled Judi's classes and vice versa, as some discos eventually began offering aerobics classes during the day. (Disco exercisers were apparently not bothered by inhaling stale cigarette smoke and cologne as they sweated.) The new genre of disco music invigorated aerobics classes across the country with its bumping beats. Disco deejays would come to influence the rhythm of aerobic dance classes, too, when they inspired fitness instructors to start teaching their classes to one continuous music track instead of breaking between songs.

Dance's popularity created a greater appreciation for women's physicality and strength. And yet, even as women demonstrated their athleticism on dance floors and marathon courses and college athletic fields, even as feminists fought against valuing women for their appearance—or perhaps in response to this progress, feminists would later argue—America's body ideals inched further out of reach for most women.

Throughout the seventies, women's magazines continued to fill their pages with advice on how to slim down—only now they enthusiastically pushed vigorous exercise as a weight-loss and figure-shaping tool along with counting calories. Pop culture began to idolize female bodies that were slim but also vaguely athletic-looking. The TV series *Wonder Woman*, which aired on ABC and then CBS from 1975 to 1979, starred Lynda Carter in a sparkly leotard, her firm physique offering a new ideal of womanhood. *Charlie's Angels*, which aired on ABC from 1976 to 1981, starred the sporty Farrah Fawcett-Majors, who became the decade's it girl. (Fawcett-Majors also helped to popularize one of the first models of women-specific running shoes, the Nike Señorita Cortez, when she wore a red, white, and blue pair in an episode of *Charlie's Angels* in 1977.) Gradually these images would raise the bar for what was considered beautiful. It was no longer enough to simply be thin. Now, pop culture suggested, a woman must also be "toned."

At the same time, the seventies saw the rise of a cultural appreciation for so-called authenticity. More women let their hair hang loose, forgoing the high-maintenance bouffant hairdos of previous decades. Makeup softened. And wardrobes became more casual.

As was true with the rise of miniskirts in the sixties, this dressing down both liberated women and reinforced physical anxieties. *Be free! Be natural! Be you!* urged women's magazines—alongside articles about dieting. In one particularly striking illustration of the era's schizophrenic treatment of women's bodies, the April 1972 issue of *Cosmopolitan* features an essay titled "Why I Hate Me," seemingly meant to enlighten women with low self-esteem, followed immediately by an ad for a full-body "slenderizing wrap," encouraging readers to regularly mummify themselves to become more attractive. Many pages later, the issue includes a strikingly feminist article about the rise of female athletes, leading editor in chief Helen Gurley Brown to write in her editor's letter: "Do you know that women are often as *physically* strong as men, so bye-bye one more myth!" (This issue also includes the magazine's first-ever nude male centerfold, featuring a hirsute, mustachioed Burt Reynolds lying naked on a bearskin rug—but that's another story for another day.)

As part of Americans' embrace of the "authentic," the decade also saw what cultural critics would call the "jeaning of America"—the cultural domination of blue jeans. Before the seventies, Americans wore loose-fitting jeans for rugged labor and play. But in the late 1960s, denim started to become fashion, as formfitting bell-bottoms became the look of the era.

In 1969, Levi Strauss & Co. released its first womenswear line, Levi's for Gals, and other denim brands followed suit. Jeans were comfortable, sure, but they also called new attention to a woman's butt, crotch, and thighs and contributed to women's desire to shape their lower bodies. One of the first Levi's for Gals print ads shows a thin but curvy woman in tight jeans sitting down in a movie theater—from behind. The copy? "The best seat in the house."

Back in Chicago, Judi Sheppard Missett was busy refining Jazz Dance for Fun and Fitness. It was now among the most popular of all Gus Giordano's offerings, and she was happy to be teaching it several times a week while continuing to dance professionally.

But Judi and Jack were growing weary of the city's brutal winters. Jack had risen through the ranks at CBS to become an on-air broadcast journalist, and after covering the tumultuous late 1960s, he was starting to burn out. He wasn't altogether disappointed when CBS laid him off during a company shake-up, though it would make finances tighter than ever for the young family. In 1972, with a new sense of freedom and a few thousand dollars to their name, they packed up and moved to San Diego, California, where Jack's brothers had settled.

During their first few months in San Diego, to pay the bills, Judi took a job as an exercise instructor at the ritzy Golden Door Health

Spa in the town of Escondido—one of the first spas to offer vigorous fitness classes—and commuted to Los Angeles for modeling and performing jobs. Jack found work as a part-time Santa Claus at a local mall, an electronics store shelf-stacker, and a graveyard shift worker at a bakery. When they weren't working, the couple explored ways for Judi to bring Jazz Dance for Fun and Fitness to their new city. Eventually she convinced a handful of local YMCAs and parks and recreation departments to let her use their facilities for a small cut of her earnings. With Jack's help as a former journalist, Judi sent out a press release to local newspapers announcing a new dance exercise program "developed in Chicago."

Judi's program initially grew through word of mouth—and it grew fast. Within a year, Judi was teaching in recreation centers and YMCAs all across the county. For publicity, she would recruit students to dance with her at local malls and fairs, farmers' markets, and beach band shells. When prospective students told her they'd love to enroll but they had no one to watch their kids, she began offering babysitting services—her sister-in-law volunteered to do the sitting for a small fee. The two women would load up the back seat of Judi's yellow Honda hatchback with toys and crayons, hop in, and take to the highway.

Around this time, while teaching a class at the La Jolla YMCA, a student asked Judi, *What do you call this thing we're doing?*

Judi reminded her: *It's Jazz Dance for Fun and Fitness!*

The student thought for a moment, then offered: *Why not call it Jazzercise?*

Judi mulled it over. The name felt fresh and cutting-edge, but still welcoming. Few fitness brands had jumped on the *-ercise* (or *-ercize*) bandwagon yet. And in the two decades since Bonnie Prudden began teaching her conditioning classes, *exercise* had gone from being a dirty word to a draw.

Judi decided to give it a go. And she had the foresight to copyright it.

———————————

By the mid-seventies, Judi was teaching twenty-five Jazzercise classes a week across Southern California. She was thrilled with her workout's success, but she was also exhausted. She had gotten thin—too thin, she thought.

Then one day she lost her voice.

When she tried to speak above a whisper, nothing came out.

Her doctor told her to see a vocal cord specialist, and the specialist told her she had developed nodules on her vocal cords. If she didn't give them a rest, he said, she could lose her voice entirely. To start, she would need to remain silent for a solid week.

Judi despaired. She had come to believe that *she*—her passion, her gift for inspiring students—was the reason her classes were so popular. "I was convinced that, unless I could be cloned, the experience couldn't be replicated," she recalled. "Who wants to think they're easily replaced?" But if she wanted her voice, and business, to survive, she needed help.

She hesitantly trained five of her most experienced and enthusiastic students to become instructors. It turned out Jazzercise as a fitness program could stand on its own.

(Judi's vocal cord ordeal would also lead to a fitness first: She and her instructors would begin teaching with microphones. In the period before wireless mikes were invented, this was a clunky practice—instructors found themselves tripping over cords during class. It wasn't until the nineties, when wireless headset mikes became available thanks to technology developed by NASA, that the practice began to feel effortless.)

In 1979, Judi incorporated her business to become Jazzercise, Inc.

She enlisted ten instructors to work out of their central office and help with everything from publicity and marketing to acquiring music records for class.

Jazzercise spread largely based on the enthusiasm of its students. Judi's original handful of instructors inspired more loyal students to become instructors, who then started more classes and inspired more students, and on and on. When instructors moved, they spread Jazzercise to new regions of the country. Because San Diego was a hub for U.S. military bases, many of Judi's early students were connected to the armed forces—which meant they moved a lot. Military families would become instrumental in spreading aerobics across the country and then around the world.

By the late seventies, Judi had landed a gig as a contributor to the morning show *Sun-Up San Diego* and was building a reputation as a national fitness expert. To shore up her expertise with science, she regularly asked exercise physiologists' advice on her methods and choreography. And in 1978, she published her first book, *Jazzercise: Rhythmic Jazz Dance Exercise, A Fun Way to Fitness*, which catapulted her to greater fame. "When was the last time you moved like a child?" she asks in the book's introduction. "Running, jumping, hopping, skipping—and felt so *good* doing it!" Jazzercise, she wrote, would "reacquaint you with your body and make your body your friend." She then encourages women to not be self-critical. "Give yourself room to grow in your attitude toward yourself and your body," she writes. "Be good to yourself by learning to become free and uninhibited in your movements!"

Capitalizing on the national interest in dance, she promises: "The fantasies you may have about being a dancer will become reality! Whenever a band strikes up the music, you will smile, enjoy yourself, and show the world you're the jazziest dancer around."

The book then offers an anatomy lesson, complete with a groovy illustrated diagram of a woman's body, and walks readers through her moves.

In many ways, *Jazzercise* reads almost like a commercial companion to *Our Bodies, Ourselves*. But like other fitness guides of the era, it veered sharply from feminist doctrine by promising a path not only to strength but also to the prospect of a lovelier, lither, more enchanting you.

"Have you seen the kicks dancers do in a chorus line?" Judi wrote. "You'll be able to do them, too, as gracefully and confidently as though you were on stage. . . . You need only the mood and the motivation, often provided by a first look in the mirror at the inches that you want to lose."

The book sold more than 400,000 copies and became an international bestseller. Judi and Jazzercisers across the country became cultural fixtures, appearing on programs from *The Phil Donahue Show* to *The Dinah Shore Show* and dancing at live events from local parades to NFL halftime productions—offering grown women who had never before performed an opportunity to feel like they were a part of something that mattered.

———————————————

By early 1982, Jazzercise had more than a thousand instructors in nearly every state and a handful of countries around the world. After her bestselling book, Judi released a workout album that went gold. Business was booming. But she found herself at a professional crossroads.

It began with a joint call from her lawyer and her accountant, who were sorry to tell her they had bad news. They had just learned that Jazzercise's business model was apparently—well, not entirely legal.

Judi had been hiring her instructors as independent contractors. For a small percentage of their gross income, she allowed them to use the Jazzercise name and provided them with choreographed routines. The problem was, this didn't meet the IRS's strict requirements for independent contractors. Judi would have to transform all of her instructors into Jazzercise employees, meaning she would be their boss, or Jazzercise franchisees, meaning they would work for themselves.

She agonized over what to do.

Eventually she told her team: *Let's go the franchise route.* It was a choice that proved crucial to the company's success. Making instructors franchisees would allow them to turn their love of Jazzercise into full-fledged careers. Judi heard the voice of her mom, who instilled in her a can-do spirit, in her ear as she took on franchising: There's always a way to get it *done.*

Judi pulled it off and was able to offer instructors an unprecedented deal. To become franchisees, instructors had to pay a mere $500 for training. From there, they were required to give the company 20 percent of their monthly gross income minus rent.

At the time "a successful Jazzercise franchisee (and most were very successful) could easily provide the owner with a net income of $75,000," Judi wrote in *Building a Business with a Beat.* This was the equivalent of around $187,500 today. By late 1982, Jazzercise was the second fastest growing franchise in the country—right behind Domino's Pizza.

To celebrate everyone's hard work, Judi organized the first Jazzercise International Instructors' Convention, held on a community college football field north of San Diego. Packed with a few thousand instructors, the event featured a surprise appearance from the hit R&B band the Spinners, who sang "Working My Way Back to You" while Judi led the crowd through spirited choreography. For the grand finale, Judi danced to the *Rocky III* anthem "Eye of the Tiger" while a 200-pound tiger named Asia "prowled across the stage" behind her. At the end, a plane appeared overhead and sky-wrote *JAZZERCISE.*

Across America, local aerobics queens began to build mini empires of their own. Some had invented original dance workouts in the sixties. Most notably, a former University of California–Berkeley pompom girl named Jacki Sorensen had introduced America to the term *aerobic dancing* in 1969—the same year Judi created Jazzercise—and launched a booming fitness business that offered classes from coast to coast. Other aerobics entrepreneurs built on what Judi, Jacki, and earlier fitness pioneers had started. Judi and Jacki Sorensen were "pilot fish at the nose end of a large school of women," writes Daniel Kunitz in *Lift: Fitness Culture, from Naked Greeks and Acrobats to Jazzercise and Ninja Warriors*, and throughout the seventies, aerobic dance spread "on tendrils sent out by these women."

The Atlanta area had Arden Zinn, who had spent time traveling with Bonnie Prudden to demonstrate her exercises while Bonnie lectured to crowds. Zinn created a dance exercise program called Ardenics and opened a chain of studios throughout the South. Her protégée was a woman named Martha Pipkin, who in 1972 launched Shape Up with Martha in Memphis, Tennessee. Over the next five years, Pipkin grew the business to include fifty instructors teaching a hundred classes. In the Northeast, there was Nancy Strong, who had been one of Bonnie's neighbors in Westchester. In 1978 she launched Aerobic Slimnastics in Connecticut and eventually oversaw more than two hundred instructors in the tristate area. The West had Sheila Cluff, who starred in a fitness TV show in New York and Vermont in the late sixties, before moving to California, where she taught Cardio-Vascular Dancing. Eventually, *aerobics* became a catchall term for these dance-based cardiovascular workouts.

While the aerobics world was dominated by women, it would also see the stratospheric ascent of one savvy male entrepreneur: Richard Simmons. The flamboyant Louisiana-born guru opened his first fitness studio in Los Angeles in the mid-seventies—the Anatomy Asylum—and quickly attracted a devoted following. He marketed his studios as welcoming spaces for women (and men) who were not already "slim and trim" and might feel self-conscious dancing among Hollywood's throngs of professionally beautiful people. He frequently referred to himself as a "former fatty."

From coast to coast, women who had grown up believing it was unladylike to sweat, many of whom did not consider themselves "athletic" and had found any excuse to skip gym class as girls, began to change their minds about exercise. Most initially sought out aerobics because it promised a slimmer, more conventionally beautiful physique. A physique that would look good in tight bell-bottoms. A physique embodied by the pretty woman teaching the class. But while the promise of cosmetic transformation might have gotten women in the door, they stuck with aerobic dancing because of how it made them *feel*. Because as feminist scholars have pointed out: As women become more physically competent, they change.

Aerobics classes gave women more energy and strength. They improved women's cardiovascular health. They offered women an emotional release and social support and a safe space to connect with their bodies. They brought women joy.

While researching this book, I interviewed aerobics instructors across the country who began teaching as young women and are now in their seventies and older, and most described the workout as a revelation. Jean Buchanan, now in her late eighties, started taking Jacki Sorensen's Aerobic Dancing when she was forty-four. Growing up, she had been taught, like many women of her generation, that vigorous exercise would make a woman's uterus "drop." After she lost her son to cancer, however, she signed up for Jacki's classes in her then-hometown of Austin, Texas, to cope with her grief, as well as to lose the weight she had gained from stress. Through aerobics, "I became a different person," she told me. "A stronger, more confident person." She eventually became an Aerobic Dancing instructor—and still teaches as of this writing in her current home of Overland Park, Kansas.

Aerobics also provided many women with lifelong friends. "We experience *life* together," longtime Jazzercise instructor Nancy Brady told Judi Sheppard Missett for her most recent book. "We've gone through marriages, divorces, births, deaths, cancers, autism, and losing weight together. The workout is the foundation of how we all met, but the relationships we've made while doing the workout is what makes us a family."

For many women, aerobics served as a gateway sport, giving them the confidence to try physical activities that had previously seemed intimidating. This proved true for my mom. In the eighties, her experience in aerobics class convinced her to start jogging—she and a few close friends trained for several half-marathons together. She also took up tennis and began playing on competitive teams.

But it would be a long time before women beyond America's white middle and upper classes would have the opportunity to experience these benefits in large numbers. While aerobics teachers in the seventies advertised a "come one, come all" approach, systemic racism and income inequality continued to make it difficult for women of color to participate. When they did, they had to navigate the potential discomfort of being the only person of color in the room. (Archival photos of Jazzercise in its early years depict an almost entirely white customer base.)

Throughout the decade, some YMCAs and fitness centers in Black communities would eventually begin offering aerobics classes, and Black media would advocate for the workout. *Essence* ran its first coverage of aerobic activity in January 1976, in a feature titled simply "Exercise." The two-page spread gave a broad introduction to the benefits of regular movement, including dance.

"We all like to think that we are physically fit," it begins. "After all, we are active. We work full days, cook, wash dishes, launder clothing, buy groceries, *drive the car*. Believing that we are really active, we proceed through life, picking up a pound here, a spread there and a dimpling that is anything but adorable. In truth we are likely out of shape. Exercise is the way in." The magazine continues: "Exercise helps us attain mastery over our bodies."

Pioneering young women of color who grew up reading articles like this one would, in the decades that followed, be inspired to launch careers in fitness, blazing an important and overdue path for the Black community to cultivate health and strength.

The Southern California–based aerobics pioneer Gilda Marx had spent most of her life in a leotard, first as a professional dancer and then as a fitness entrepreneur. One of this country's earliest aerobics evangelists, Gilda—along with her husband, Bob Marx, son of comic legend Gummo Marx—ran a popular fitness studio in West Los Angeles called Body Design by Gilda, housed in a Century City penthouse. The studio was light and airy, with huge windows and floor-to-ceiling mirrors.

From the start, the studio attracted a glittery clientele, from Barbra Streisand to Playboy Bunnies and the Bond girl Britt Ekland—yes, the same Bond girl who introduced Lydia Bach to Lotte Berk. But her influence would extend beyond the rich and famous when she embarked on a quest to transform the era's universal exercise uniform: She wanted to build a better leotard.

Gilda appreciated how leotards allowed her to move with ease. But it bugged her that unless you were built like a prepubescent ballerina, leotards weren't always comfortable—or flattering.

Despite Bonnie Prudden's efforts with Capezio to revamp leotards for the masses in the fifties, they hadn't changed that much since their introduction by French acrobat Jules Léotard in the nineteenth century. Léotard's initial claim to fame was inventing the flying trapeze—he's the "daring young man" of the famous song. He wore the stretchy suit to "fly through the air with the greatest of ease," and in time, dancers embraced it, too. By the 1930s, leotards dyed pink or black were dancers' rehearsal wear of choice.

Because the leotards of mid-century America were made of natural fiber blends, however, they rode up in places they should stay down and sagged in places they should stay up. Gilda knew there had to be a better design—one that supported, flattered, and fit properly. "I wanted to create a beautiful garment that would inspire my students to want to exercise," she wrote. One that was "flexible, functional and fantastically glamorous"—a "uniform for exercise success."

The key, she would discover, was in one of the DuPont chemical company's newest synthetic fibers: Lycra. The company had spent decades developing Lycra in a quest to design a more comfortable girdle, but the fiber's triumph would come not from restricting women's bodies but from setting them free.

The story of how DuPont came to outfit not only Gilda Marx and her students but active women the world over is one of American social progress itself. It begins in the 1920s, when the Delaware-based chemical giant—which had spent its first century producing gunpowder—underwent a dramatic rebranding. In an effort to distance itself from the carnage of World War I, the company began to market itself as one that existed primarily to serve women.

"During the explosives period, Dupont's customers had been male, and its orientation and identity masculine," writes the anthropologist Kaori O'Connor, who in the early twenty-first century gained rare access to the company's archives and in 2011 published an investigation into the birth of Lycra. But in the 1920s and 1930s, recognizing that wives now had "asking power" in their homes, it saw pleasing women as a lucrative business strategy. "Better Things for Better Living, Through Chemistry" became its catchphrase.

DuPont delivered on this promise when it introduced women to nylon pantyhose.

From the 1920s through the 1960s, wearing stockings was a requirement of womanhood—everyone did it, regardless of social class. But after surveying women about stockings' shortcomings, DuPont set out to create an alternative to silk that was sheer and durable but "stable in price and more certain of supply." In 1939, its scientists had a *eureka!* moment when they successfully grew the fiber that would become nylon in a test tube. The first nylon stockings went on sale in May 1940; they were so popular, many shops saw riots of women attempting to get their hands on them.

From there, DuPont set its sights on an even more ambitious prize: the almighty girdle.

In the 1940s, as was true with pantyhose, every American woman over the age of around twelve wore a girdle. "In the period when Dupont was casting around for new synthetic fiber opportunities, it was taken for granted that a woman should not appear in public, and hardly in private, unless she was wearing a girdle," writes O'Connor. Girdles were a "hallmark of respectability" and a prerequisite for looking good in clothes. "The most disapproved-of natural features for which the girdle was seen as the corrective were fat, sag, bulge, and jiggle."

But the experience of wearing a girdle was hellish. This was partly due to the fabric, which was made from rubber-covered thread. "There is no parallel in modern textiles to the stiffness of rubberized girdle fabric, which compressed the body in a way that would now be considered intolerable," writes O'Connor. She continues:

Getting into a girdle was a complex operation, described to me as "a struggle" and "murder" by women now in their seventies and eighties. This was the case even if the wearer was of normal weight or even thin, because to be effective the rubberized girdle had to fit very tightly, and fastening it up was awkward. If the girdle had hook-and-eye fastenings, the flesh had to be pinched, pushed and prodded out of harm's way as the edges were pulled together and fastened hook by hook. Zipper fastenings were also challenging—it was difficult to keep the edges together and pull up the zip at the same time, and in the process the flesh often got pinched painfully. . . . Once encased in the girdle, normal body movements like bending and sitting became awkward, eating was uncomfortable, and performing basic body functions could become problematic. One woman recalled: "They used to say we ladies took a long time in the powder room. We weren't powdering our noses. We were struggling with our girdles." Once a girdle was removed or lowered, it was almost impossible to get it back on, and many women remembered having to "hold on" until they got home.

When DuPont surveyed American women about their dream innovations, women consistently asked for more comfortable girdles. Given that nearly *any* innovation would improve on the current models, the company saw the potential for massive earnings.

And so, in the early 1940s, its engineers embarked on a multimillion-dollar effort to create the perfect sturdy but stretchy—or *spandex*, as engineers began to call it, which was an anagram of *expands*—fiber with which to offer women more forgiving figure shapers.

Fifteen years later, a DuPont chemist named Joe Shivers revealed what he and his colleagues referred to internally as Fiber K. Shivers filed a patent application, and after more testing, by gosh, the men knew they'd done it. Fiber K "stretched and snapped back into place like rubber, but unlike rubber was resistant to deterioration caused by perspiration, cosmetic oils and lotions." It could be dyed and machine-washed and -dried. It was lighter than rubberized thread but had much more restraining power. The company officially named it Lycra.

For the debut of Lycra girdles in 1960, DuPont launched a flashy promotional campaign, running full-page ads in women's magazines from *Vogue* to *Good Housekeeping* with the tagline "at last." *At last, a girdle that lets you put in an 8-hour day—controlled but comfortable!* one read. *At last, a girdle that lets you golf, bowl, ski—do any sport in utter comfort!* another promised.

At first Lycra girdles were a hit, as demand outran supply.

Then a curious thing happened.

Despite the fact that the first massive wave of baby boomers were becoming teenagers—the age when most women began to purchase figure shapers—girdle sales started to fall. DuPont and the rest of corporate America had assumed that the young boomer women would shop and dress like their mothers. Instead, they were faced with the "youthquake" and miniskirts and Mary Quant.

Throughout the sixties, DuPont poured resources into trying to keep women in girdles. Perhaps it was merely the word *girdle* to which teens were averse? In 1968, the company helped launch an item it called a "form-persuasive garment," aimed specifically at the teen market. No luck. Worse, women of *all* ages started to reject their girdles. When, in 1968, the president of the undergarment manufacturer Playtex learned that his own wife had thrown away her girdles, the end seemed nigh.

Despite popular legend, few women in the late sixties and early seventies actually burned their bras, but most did trash their girdles. "'Getting rid of the girdle' emerged as a significant cultural moment, in every sense a defining act of 'emancipation,'" writes O'Connor. "Its abandonment was political action on the personal level, an act of liberation through stuff."

By 1975, girdle sales were half of what they had been a decade earlier.

With American women now moving about happily un-girdled, the country began to accumulate warehouses full of unwanted girdle fabric, including rolls upon rolls of a shiny new Antron nylon/Lycra blend dyed a rainbow of vibrant colors.

Gradually, small professional dancewear manufacturers and seamstresses began to snatch it up to make garments that, they discovered, "hugged the body and moved with it in a way that had never been possible before."

But it was Gilda Marx who would bring Antron nylon/Lycra leotards to the masses.

In her quest to design the perfect aerobics uniform, one that was both functional and fashionable, Gilda teamed up with a manufacturer who until then had specialized in car seat upholstery. With her home temporarily converted into a leotard laboratory, she experimented with different Lycra blends until she found her holy grail.

In 1975, Gilda introduced the Flexatard, a nylon-Lycra blend leotard with all the support of a girdle and none of the cultural baggage. Flexatards came in long-sleeved, cap-sleeve, and spaghetti strap versions. And they came in dark, chic colors—red and burgundy and navy—and later, yellow and peach and green and raspberry.

She opened a small boutique in her penthouse exercise studio and began selling Flexatards to students, who served as a kind of focus group for her products, providing instant feedback on the designs. She was buoyed by the response from her celebrity clients.

"One day I looked at the back of my class and saw Bette Midler with arms, legs, and everything flying," she wrote in her 1984 fitness book, *Body by Gilda*. "She was having a wonderful time"—and wearing a Flexatard. "After the class a panting Divine Miss M bounced up to me and said, 'I absolutely adored this workout and this leotard is great. It is the first leotard that was ever able to support my chest.' To a leotard designer, that was the ultimate challenge and the ultimate compliment."

Gilda and Bob incorporated as Flexatard, Inc., and before long, women in aerobics classes across the country would be wearing her garments. (Those colorful leotards Judi Sheppard Missett wore in her *Let's Jazzercise* video? Flexatards!) Dancewear giants Capezio and Danskin got in on the game, too, and began making their own colorful Lycra-blend attire for aerobic dancers.

When anthropologist Kaori O'Connor interviewed women about their memories of slipping into Lycra leotards and leggings for the first time, they told her it felt exhilarating. The fabric bonded women exercisers, they said, by serving as a kind of collective aerobics uniform that "seemed to free the body and hold it, cover it and yet expose it."

Perhaps most remarkably, many women told her they appreciated that the new workout wear showed their sweat. After all, sweating was now the point.

Gilda's Flexatards were a "harbinger," writes O'Connor. By the early eighties, Lycra leotards and leggings would burst out of the studio and onto the street, as Gilda and other designers introduced tops, skirts, and shorts that allowed women to come and go from aerobics class without having to change. Leotards also became popular among women who didn't exercise but liked their fresh, edgy "fashion look."

Remarkably, in "a striking example of cultural blindness, few in the mainstream seemed to realize that the beloved 'new' stretch fiber was the very stuff of which the hated and rejected girdle had been made," writes O'Connor. "Or that leotards and leggings looked identical to the new all-in-one foundation garments."

In 1984 alone, American women purchased 21 million leotards.

The rise of the leotard represented another paradigm shift in the way women viewed their physicality. "Lycra became the second skin for a new life in which self-confidence would be rooted in women and their bodies, not in rules, dress codes, wearing clothes that were 'appropriate' for age or social status, and especially not in wearing girdles," writes O'Connor. "What had been the ultimate fiber of control now became the defining fiber of freedom."

By the dawn of the eighties, aerobic dancing had risen to become a full-fledged cultural movement, touching nearly every aspect of American life—from how women spent their leisure time and money to how they dressed. In the years that followed, its popularity would spur scores of Americans to enter the fitness industry, transforming exercise's role in women's lives in ways both constructive and destructive. New varieties of aerobics classes would move beyond Judi Sheppard Missett's original vision of emotional release to become a vehicle through which women were more explicitly encouraged to strive for a standard of physical perfection unattainable for most, creating a thorny landscape to navigate in the pursuit of strength and happiness.

Jazzercise, meanwhile, continued to grow throughout the eighties, and Judi's star continued to rise. After Jazzercisers danced for a TV audience of millions at the Los Angeles Olympics, they were invited to perform at the 1986 rededication of the Statue of Liberty, a $6 million extravaganza held at Giants Stadium. That same year, President Ronald Reagan honored Judi as one of the country's "top woman entrepreneurs," and she would go on to receive an inaugural lifetime achievement award from the President's Council on Physical Fitness and Sports alongside honorees including Bonnie Prudden, Jack LaLanne, and Dr. Ken Cooper.

Most remarkably: The company is still going strong as of this writing. As the wider fitness culture evolved throughout the nineties and aughts, so did Jazzercise, rebranding and expanding its offerings to include strength-training and high-intensity interval training (HIIT) and an on-demand streaming service. (Judi's look evolved, too: You can track the fashion and hair trends of the seventies through today by studying her archives alone.)

Jazzercise is now largely run by Judi's daughter, company president Shanna Missett Nelson. In 2019 it had 8,500 franchisees, and on any given day, its instructors were teaching 70,000 students around the world. The company also boasted the largest and longest retention of customers in the fitness industry. A full *half* of Jazzercise students have attended classes for a decade or more.

When we spoke at the beginning of the COVID-19 pandemic, Judi, then seventy-six, was concerned for Jazzercise's future but cautiously optimistic. "We've gone through so many transitions, over fifty years, we will weather the storm," she told me. "I'm not sure how, but we will. It's teaching us patience, it's teaching us discipline, and it's teaching us about kindness. I think if you can learn from those things, you are going to be far better off."

As for Gilda Marx—in the late seventies, Gilda and Bob also experimented with franchising. Eventually there were more than two dozen Body Design by Gilda studios in cities from Los Angeles to New York, and, according to Gilda's 1984 book, her instructors taught "hundreds of thousands" of students. But in 1985, Gilda decided to shutter her studios and focus entirely on her fashion lines, which she grew into a multimillion-dollar business.

In the mid-eighties, Gilda collaborated with DuPont to introduce a new fiber called CoolMax—billed as "lightweight, soft and non-chafing"—and she would coin the term *breathable* to describe fabrics that aired out parts of the body that tended to sweat. She would also launch a line of garments that would surely have made the mid-century DuPont men's heads explode: aerobics leotards designed to prevent bacterial yeast infections. "Gilda Marx just solved one of your most intimate exercise problems," declared a 1989 ad for the leotards in *Vogue*. "Working out usually involves working up a sweat. But unfortunately, the heat and perspiration that go along with a good workout can cause an unhealthy environment for one of the most delicate areas of your body." The new line was, according to the ad, "just what the doctor ordered."

Products like these would, in the early nineties, inspire Oprah Winfrey to tell her legions of fans: "I personally love Gilda because she understands a woman's body."

But beyond revolutionizing women's workout wear, beyond helping to create the aesthetic of the eighties, and beyond ushering in the contemporary era of athleisure, Gilda would also inspire one of her most famous celebrity clients to try her own hand at running an exercise business.

Her name was Jane Fonda.

CHAPTER 5

Burn

Discipline is liberation.

—Martha Graham

A good many dramatic situations begin with screaming.

—Barbarella, *Barbarella*, 1968

By the dawn of the eighties, America had a self-esteem problem. The upheaval of the past two decades had shattered any illusion that the country was impervious. The economic recession was taking its toll on the nation's well-being. And President Jimmy Carter had developed a reputation, fairly or not, for being a weak and waffling leader.

Carter's apparent weakness was underscored when, during a publicized 6.2-mile run at Camp David in 1979, the president collapsed at the 4-mile mark, falling into the arms of two aides. His critics seized on this very public physical fail as metaphor, notes historian Shelly McKenzie in *Getting Physical*: here was a guy who couldn't go the distance.

When onetime Hollywood screen idol and former California governor Ronald Reagan campaigned for president, it was no coincidence that he tried to project an image of strength—particularly since, at age sixty-nine, he would be the oldest incoming president in U.S. history up to that point. Reagan, a master of self-presentation, was often shown chopping wood and clearing brush at his California ranch. The president-to-be told voters: *We are the greatest country on earth, and I will lift us back up to our natural place at the top of the global food chain.* He made downtrodden Americans feel like winners again.

Reagan would continue to cultivate an image of physical strength throughout his presidency. After surviving an assassination attempt in 1981, he took up weightlifting and boasted that his chest had grown two inches. He showed off his bulging biceps in national magazines. In time, he would help to make the eighties the decade of the so-called power physique, writes McKenzie, as "muscles became a symbol of the new national toughness."

The early evangelism of Bonnie Prudden and the pioneers who followed her was now paying off. Nearly half of Americans said they exercised regularly, according to a 1977 Gallup poll, including a striking 45 percent of women. Women were jogging and aerobic dancing, as well as cycling and skiing and playing tennis. They were taking pride in their physicality. They were sold.

So when one of the most admired women in the world—herself a Hollywood movie star—started advocating for fitness, America paid attention. For women who already exercised, she offered affirmation; for non-exercisers, she gave them the push they needed to start sweating. She told women to "go for the burn," and her message caught fire.

Jane Fonda offered women the ultimate promise: Do like me, and you can *be* like me.

It's understandable that many people assume a book about the history of women's fitness would begin here. Jane Fonda's popularity was so vast, her impact on women's exercise habits so profound, she has been engraved into the collective consciousness as the beginning of women's workout culture, full stop. As former Body Design by Gilda studio manager and aerobics pioneer Ken Alan told me: "I think of women's fitness history as BJ and AJ. Before Jane and After Jane."

————————

Who was Jane Fonda in 1979, when she opened her original aerobics studio in Beverly Hills? To the public, Jane, then forty-two years old, was the woman with everything. After a decade of controversy surrounding her activism, Jane had a newly flourishing acting career. She was stunningly gorgeous, defying decades-old stereotypes about women of a certain age. She was a devoted mother and wife. *Redbook*'s readers had recently voted her a woman they most admired. But in private, she was searching and stumbling and struggling to build a life that would make her feel whole and happy.

Born Lady Jayne Seymour Fonda in 1937, the future superstar grew up a sad little girl in the mountains of Bel Air. Her early life was lonely and reckless and traumatic, shaped by her famous father, the actor Henry Fonda, who deprived his daughter of any affection or affirmation, and a remote, mentally ill mother. "All my life I [have] been [my] father's daughter, trapped in a Greek drama, like Athena, who sprang fully formed from the head of her father, Zeus—disciplined, driven," Jane wrote in her memoir, *My Life So Far*. "I learned that love was earned through perfection."

Jane's mother, Frances, had wanted a baby boy, and Jane felt her disappointment—particularly after her brother, the actor Peter Fonda, was born and Frances made it clear he was her favorite. But Jane was most scarred by her father's seeming indifference. She began to wish she had been a boy, too. She cut off her long braids and dressed in jeans and T-shirts to roam the rocky hills around her family's sprawling compound.

From her earliest days, Jane had a deep psychological need to transform herself, wrote the late journalist Patricia Bosworth, who knew Jane for forty years before she wrote her friend's biography, *Jane Fonda: The Private Life of a Public Woman.* "It was the start of countless self-inventions in the vain hope of being recognized, acknowledged, and noticed by her father."

When Jane was eleven years old, Henry Fonda accepted a role starring in the play *Mister Roberts* on Broadway, and the family moved to Greenwich, Connecticut, a short train ride from New York City. While starring in the play, her father fell in love with a stage manager's sister, Susan Blanchard. Susan was the stepdaughter of the great Broadway lyricist Oscar Hammerstein II, and she was only seven years older than Jane. Henry's marriage to Frances had been crumbling for many years as Frances was gripped more and more by bipolar disorder—a reality he called a "bore."

Henry's request for a divorce sent Frances over the edge. While in the care of a psychiatric institute in New York's Hudson Valley, Frances used a small, smuggled-in razor to slit her throat in a bathroom.

Henry Fonda and their grandmother Sophie would tell Jane and Peter that their mother had died of a heart attack. Jane would discover the truth about her mother's death a few months later, when she read about it in a celebrity gossip magazine.

In 1950, when Jane was fourteen, her father and grandmother sent her to the Emma Willard boarding school in Upstate New York. It was a year after her mother's death, and she had "perfected an air of supreme indifference," wrote Bosworth. Still, Jane liked being in the company of other young women—growing up, her happiest times had been spent with other adventurous little girls, exploring and riding horses and playing games.

But Jane's years at boarding school would also mark the beginning of a decades-long struggle with eating disorders. Her mother had been a compulsive dieter, obsessed with her weight and warning her young daughter that a woman must be thin to be desirable. She would tell her, "Lady, if I gain any extra weight, I'm going to cut it off with a knife!"

Her insecurities were compounded by the fact that Henry Fonda had "an obsession with women being thin," Jane wrote. "Once I hit adolescence, the only time my father ever referred to how I looked was when he thought I was too fat," she wrote. "The truth is that I was never fat. But that wasn't what mattered. For a girl trying to please others, what mattered was how I saw myself—how I'd learned to see myself: through others' judgmental, objectifying eyes."

And so, at school, Jane made slimness her number one goal. "Starting my freshman year at Emma Willard, being very thin assumed dominance over good hair in the hierarchy of what really mattered," she wrote. As a young teen, she bought chewing gum packed with tapeworm eggs after seeing it advertised in a magazine. It didn't work, she wrote, but "anything that would allow me to get thin without having to do something active seemed attractive."

During Jane's sophomore year at boarding school, her new best friend, Carol, introduced her to the concept of binging and purging. Carol had been inspired after learning in history class about the ancient Roman tradition of gorging on food and then throwing it up. Neither teen had heard of bulimia, nor did they know that it could harm them or become an addiction. "Aha," Jane remembers thinking, naively, "here's a way to *not* have our cake and eat it, too."

After boarding school, Jane enrolled at Vassar College in Poughkeepsie, New York, where she drank too much, got hooked on amphetamines, and failed her exams. After two years, she dropped out and eventually moved to New York City to pursue an acting career.

Jane had begun to dabble with acting in high school, appearing in school productions. She was drawn to theater because it offered a way to connect with her father. But she also found it provided some relief from the constant ache she felt inside. Acting allowed her to step out of herself and become someone else for a while.

In New York, Jane sought out work as a fashion model to pay for acting classes and appeared on the cover of nearly every major magazine, from *Life* to *Vogue* to *Ladies' Home Journal*. The modeling did nothing to boost her confidence; it only made her feel even more self-conscious. Along with bingeing and purging and taking amphetamines, Jane now began taking diuretic pills. As her weight plunged, she would spend hours critiquing her face and body in the mirror.

Jane landed her first on-screen role in a 1960 romantic comedy called *Tall Story*, opposite Tony Perkins. Starring in a film was not quite what Jane had imagined. It was glamorous, yes, but the experience also subjected her to more scrutiny. When Jack Warner, head of the Warner Bros. studio, saw Jane's makeup tests, he and the film's director suggested that after shooting wrapped, "Jane might consider having her jaw broken and reset, and her back teeth pulled to create a more chiseled look—specifically, one that emulated the sunken cheekbones that were the hallmark of Suzy Parker, the supermodel of that time," wrote Bosworth. They also suggested she start wearing falsies.

But in January 1961, Jane auditioned for and was accepted as a lifetime member of New York's legendary Actors Studio. Her career was off and running.

In her late twenties, Jane married the French film director Roger Vadim, and he was the driving force behind her star-making role in the late sixties sci-fi camp classic, *Barbarella*. At thirty, she got pregnant. Her pregnancy spanned 1968—that crucial and tumultuous year in American history, when both Martin Luther King Jr. and Robert Kennedy were assassinated, and anti–Vietnam War protesters clashed with police near the Democratic National Convention in Chicago. It was during her pregnancy that Jane felt her first urges toward activism.

Jane was the first to admit that she had never been especially politically aware. But she found that while she was pregnant, she was like a sponge—more attuned than ever before to the wider world. She also began to see America through the eyes of the French (she and her husband were living outside Paris at the time), and she grew increasingly frustrated and appalled.

A friend gave her a copy of *The Village of Ben Suc*, which detailed American atrocities in Vietnam. "I closed the book," she later wrote. "I knew that something fundamental in the general area of my heart had exploded and blown me wide open." She wanted to do something—but what?

Over the next few years, Jane felt herself growing further away from Roger Vadim, owing partly to his many vices. Jane was the primary earner in their home, and Vadim gambled away what she made. He drank too much and too often. He had convinced Jane to open their bed to a steady stream of women, many of them high-priced call girls, whom Jane was responsible for soliciting. Jane tried to convince herself she had become sexually enlightened, but deep down the arrangement fueled her insecurities.

In 1970, Jane moved back to California. She cut her long blond Barbarella locks into a short androgynous bob. And in 1973, she divorced Vadim and moved more toward the full-throated activism that had been simmering inside of her for years.

By the time Jane found her activist calling, the anti–Vietnam War movement of the sixties had lost steam. The war had raged on for sixteen years and claimed the lives of more than 50,000 American servicemen and hundreds of thousands of North Vietnamese and Viet Cong fighters; the total tally of Vietnamese lives lost on the ground was nearing 2 million. And even within the peace movement, there was division. But activists were hopeful that with her immense fame, Jane could help to unite and reignite the movement.

President Nixon began to see Jane's political potential, too, and he and his FBI director, J. Edgar Hoover, began to surveil and attempt to intimidate her. "What in the world is the matter with Jane Fonda?" Nixon is heard saying in 1971 on one of the notorious Nixon tapes. "I feel so sorry for Henry Fonda, who's a nice man. She's a great actress. She looks pretty. But boy, she's often on the wrong track."

The most famous and infamous moment in Jane's antiwar activism makes the story of her eventual transformation into a wildly popular fitness icon even more remarkable. In May 1972, Jane traveled to Vietnam to see the horrors America had wrought on the country with her own eyes. During a two-week tour, she bonded with Vietnamese emissaries and spoke on Radio Hanoi, pleading with U.S. troops not to drop bombs.

Finally, on the last day of her trip, her Vietnamese hosts arranged for her to visit an antiaircraft installation on the outskirts of Hanoi. The plan didn't sit right with her, but they insisted. When Jane arrived, someone put a military helmet on her head and asked her to climb into the gunner's seat. She reluctantly agreed and smiled, as cameras snapped. Then the panic set in. "Oh my God," she thought. "It's going to look like I was trying to shoot down U.S. planes!" When Nixon loyalists caught wind of what happened, they lambasted her as a traitor, dubbing her Hanoi Jane.

She regrets the incident to this day, writing, "That two-minute lapse of sanity will haunt me until I die."

In the years after she left Roger Vadim, Jane had many lovers. She dated her *Klute* costar, Donald Sutherland, who was equally devoted to activism. But she didn't see how she could be married to her work and another man at the same time. Then she met Tom Hayden, the man who would provide the unlikeliest of paths to the Workout.

Tom was a celebrity in his own right. He had been a radical leftist hero of the sixties peace movement and a leader of the protests at the 1968 Democratic Convention in Chicago. His role in these protests, which descended into violent clashes with the police, led President Nixon to charge him with conspiracy—he was one of the seven defendants in the infamous trial of the Chicago Seven. But unlike many of his radical peers, he hadn't given up the cause. He was still fighting to end the Vietnam War.

Jane and Tom had crossed paths a few times on the road, but nothing came of it. Then, in 1972, Tom attended a talk Jane gave on the horrific impact of the war in Vietnam. Afterward, he looked for her backstage and suggested they team up some time. He was living in a run-down apartment in Venice, California, teaching classes about the culture and people of Vietnam at a nearby university.

Tom wasn't exactly a matinee idol.* He was scruffy and pockmarked, with a bulbous nose, but he had an impish charm. "Putting his hand on my knee, he said he'd also just finished his own slideshow and that 'I'd like to show it to you sometime,'" Jane wrote in her memoir. "At least I think that's what he said. An electric charge had gone right through me, and all I was thinking about at that moment was his hand on my knee."

Jane fell hard. "I wanted a man in my life I could love . . . but it had to be someone who could inspire me, teach me, lead me, not be afraid of me." In Tom, she believed she had found that man. She had

---

* Some critics raised an eyebrow at director Aaron Sorkin's decision to cast actor Eddie Redmayne as Tom Hayden in his 2020 film *The Trial of the Chicago 7*, among other quibbles with the movie.

heard he could be controlling and power-hungry—but he seemed genuinely enthralled by her.*

The following year, Jane and Tom Hayden married. They had a baby boy together, whom they named Troy. And they moved into a drab two-family house on a dingy street in Santa Monica. Tom believed true activists should not live with privilege, but with the people. Hayden felt strongly that they should not own a dishwasher or a washing machine. For a decade, the couple slept on a mattress on the floor.

Throughout the seventies, Jane threw herself into helping make Tom's political dreams a reality. He had been mostly out of the public eye since his conspiracy trial, but he still had big ambitions. They both believed he could be president someday. "Jane set out to make Tom Hayden visible after a long eclipse," wrote Bosworth, working with Hollywood press agents to reintroduce Tom to the world as a moderate family-friendly Democrat.

Around this time, Tom Hayden found a fan in César Chávez, the legendary labor leader and civil rights activist. Chávez advised Tom that if he wanted to get elected to public office, he would first need to build a movement—a "machine for the people."

Tom followed his new friend's advice. Together with Jane, he launched the grassroots Campaign for Economic Democracy, or CED, to move power "out of the hands of the superrich and the corporations, into the hands of people, the way it should be in a democracy," as well as to promote liberal causes and candidates, including solar energy, nuclear disarmament, and women's rights. There was just one problem: money—or more precisely, the lack of it.

---

* Jane Fonda wasn't the only fitness guru to be romantically linked to a member of the Chicago Seven. Mimi Leonard, sister of The Bar Method founder Burr Leonard and a barre studio owner herself, was married to Yippie co-founder and radical activist Jerry Rubin for fourteen years.

How would they fund CED? Building the kind of political army they envisioned would require loads of cash. "I was making one or more movies a year by now," Jane wrote, "most quite successful, and every premiere would be a benefit for CED. Still, we worried about being able to sustain the work."

The answer, it turned out, was "staring her right in the face."

Throughout Jane's transformations, one thing had remained consistent: She was obsessed with being super-thin. She achieved this goal mostly through acts of self-destruction—starvation, bulimia, a dependence on diuretics and stimulants.

From boarding school through her years as a young actress in New York through her marriage to Vadim and now Tom, Jane had binged and purged. At times she was also anorexic, eating only a soft-boiled egg and spinach daily. Her eating disorders and addictions made her feel perpetually irritable, preoccupied, and exhausted.

But there was one activity that actually made her feel good: ballet.

Jane discovered ballet in her early twenties. Her boyfriend at the time was a professional dancer, and he introduced her to one of his favorite studios in New York City. Jane took to ballet immediately. She was no great talent, but she was double-jointed and could do many of the moves reasonably well. She loved the discipline ballet required, and she began to appreciate the way the physical exertion made her feel. Ballet classes, she wrote in her memoir, offered a path to "keeping at least a tenuous connection to my body."

Throughout the sixties and seventies, Jane took ballet compulsively. She took classes in New York and France and in towns across the United States while on location making films. She would go to class at four o'clock in the morning, before shooting began, or at night after a marathon day on set.

Beyond making her feel centered and strong and in control, Jane also loved that ballet offered a reliable way to remain as lithe as possible. In the days after giving birth to Vanessa, Jane wanted to lose weight "immediately" and began doing ballet pliés in the hospital bathroom. She started hemorrhaging and had to stay in the hospital for an additional week.

In 1978, while filming *The China Syndrome*, a drama about a nuclear power plant leak that eerily preceded the historic accident on Three Mile Island, Jane remained committed as ever to ballet. Then she tripped on the set and broke her foot.

She was constantly fracturing her feet throughout her thirties; her eating disorders had weakened her bones. This time, though, the injury was bad enough that she would have to give up ballet for a while. "What to do?" she wrote. "I had to get in shape for my next movie, *California Suite*, in which I had to appear in a bikini."

By now, her father, Henry Fonda, was married to his fifth (and final) wife. Shirlee Fonda was a former flight attendant and model, and she was only five years older than Jane. Jane shared her predicament with Shirlee, and her stepmother told her that, when her foot had sufficiently healed, she simply *had* to check out the fabulous exercise classes she had started taking at a studio in Century City. It was run by a woman named Gilda Marx.

In June 1978, Jane made her way to the Body Design by Gilda penthouse studio. She signed up for a class taught by a popular instructor named Leni Cazden, whom her stepmother had recommended, and hoped for the best.

Leni was in her early thirties and projected "an enigmatic combination of aloofness and availability," according to Jane. That first day, Leni dedicated the class to the intrepid female explorer Naomi James, who had just become the second woman to sail solo around the earth. Leni had recently taken up sailing herself, and she told the class, "If she can do that, we can certainly get through this next hour and a half."

For Jane, the class was a revelation.

Like so many in the seventies, she found the experience of sweating in a room packed with other women thrilling. The class engaged her entire body, working muscles she didn't know she had. It focused on "strengthening and toning through the use of an interesting combination of repetitive movements that included, to my great pleasure, a surprising amount of ballet." The day after her first class, she was so sore she had trouble sitting down.

Jane was surprised to find herself connecting to the class's music, too. While other exercise classes at Body Design by Gilda were taught to disco, Leni's selections were more soulful—Al Green and Fleetwood Mac, Stevie Wonder and Marvin Gaye. "Up until then I had known next to nothing about current popular music," Jane wrote. "If I listened to the radio, it was to NPR for the news. Now these new sounds entered my life. I began to move to a different rhythm, becoming one of those people you see through their car windows singing and grooving to music only they can hear."

She never went back to ballet.

Jane became a regular at Body Design by Gilda and one of Leni's most loyal students. "I hated to miss even a day," she wrote. When Leni wasn't scheduled to teach, she would hire her for private sessions.

It was around this time that Jane and Tom were searching for a business to fund the Campaign for Economic Democracy. One day, when Jane was waxing rhapsodic to her stepmother about Gilda's studio and everything it offered women, Shirlee told her: "You could open a studio, too, you know."

Of course! Jane thought.

Jane asked Leni if she would be interested in launching a fitness studio with her, and Leni liked the idea. They would call their business Jane and Leni's Workout.

———————————

For a long time, Leni Cazden kept quiet about being the secret architect of a worldwide cultural phenomenon. But her workout was her masterpiece. "To be asked how I created my workout is equivalent to being asked who I am," Leni told me when we spoke in July 2020. Creating her workout—which evolved into the Jane Fonda Workout—was "a culmination of all my experience and all my training."

Before meeting Jane, Leni had lived a difficult life. She, too, had survived a mentally ill mother and a traumatic childhood in Orange County, California. Growing up in the 1950s, Leni was in and out of child protective services, and she became a self-described diehard tomboy. Eventually she found solace in an unlikely sport: roller skating. "I was pretty much on my own at a young age, and I took myself to the rink. That's where I found myself. My home life was so undisciplined, I think I was looking for discipline."

She would race, and eventually compete, in roller dancing—which was like ice dancing but on wheels. "When I was young, I was weird because I was so athletic," she told me. "But I liked being king of the mountain."

She eventually took her routines to the ice and won championships with her performances. When Leni was sixteen, she married her ice-skating partner, who was twenty years her senior. She was desperate to be free of her childhood home. Not long after, she had a daughter who died in infancy followed by a second daughter, whom she named Lauri.

By the early 1970s, Leni had split from her husband and retired from ice skating. After a few years of traveling across California as a hippie, child in tow, she eventually made her way to Los Angeles.

She needed a way to support herself and Lauri, so she began taking dance classes and adapting what she had learned on the rink for the exercise studio. Eventually she landed a job teaching dance exercise at a popular L.A. gym—the Beverly Hills Health Club for Women. Next she was hired by Richard Simmons to work at his fitness studio, Anatomy Asylum. Finally, she was scouted and hired by Gilda Marx, who was devoting more time to Flexatard Inc. and needed instructors to teach her classes.

Leni wanted to create a workout that was truly original. "If I was going to teach an exercise class, then it was going to be top-notch," she told me. "I spent hours upon hours in my living room choreographing how each and every movement would flow to the next."

Her workout was challenging. She decided to make it ninety minutes long, since that was the length of a typical dance class. And she set it to popular music. "At the time, I had only seen people use their voices, claps, and snaps to move their classes along," she said. "My whole life had been set to music and this would be no different."

At Body Design by Gilda, Leni became hugely popular. The classroom was her "utopia," and she was happier than she had ever been in her life. "Every once in a while I'd look out and see the whole room rocking, and I went, *wow*. It was very emotional for me."

When celebrities would show up to her class, Leni would at first feel a little starstruck, but then she'd get over it. "Exercise is the great equalizer," she said—it revealed stars' humanity. On Jane's first day of class, Leni remembers telling her new famous pupil to be gentle with herself and avoid the more advanced moves. Jane, she remembers, didn't listen.

As soon as Jane and Leni agreed to go into business together, they got to work. Over the next year, Leni trained Jane in the nuances of her workout, which Jane herself planned to teach a few times a week. Leni taught her how to put on leg warmers, which dancers had worn for decades to limber up their muscles, and which were now becoming part of the dance exercise aesthetic. ("Nobody knew how to wear them," said Leni. "If you want them to look cool, if you want them to flatter your leg, you've got to know where to put them.")

Leni made Jane audiocassettes with music and exercise cues so Jane could practice the workout when she was away from L.A. and on location. While filming *The Electric Horseman* with Robert Redford in Utah, Jane arranged to teach her first classes, instructing women (and a few men) who were part of the film crew in the basement of a small spa.

"The experience of teaching such a diverse group opened my eyes to a much broader array of the benefits of exercise than I had ever expected," Jane wrote. "One woman said she'd stopped needing sleeping pills. People told me they felt less stressed. Most profound, though, were the testimonials that showed how women were starting to feel differently about themselves—empowered."

Meanwhile, Leni found a light-filled space for sale on an unassuming stretch of Robertson Boulevard in Beverly Hills. Jane liked it and invested $100,000 in renovations. Leni began working with an architect to convert it into a fitness studio with three classrooms lined in floor-to-ceiling mirrors. Leni also began scouting for instructors. "Everything was coming together quickly," she told me.

In the weeks before the studio was set to open in September 1979, Jane and Tom went on a seventy-five-city tour across the country—Jane called it a "blitz pilgrimage"—to raise money for CED and speak out against nuclear weapons. The tour began with a massive rally in New York City's Battery Park, where, Bosworth wrote, Tom declared that "There will be a nuclear Armageddon unless something is done!"

Jane visited six more cities on her own, where she encouraged crowds of women—particularly secretaries and clerical workers—to organize and fight for equality. The plight of underpaid working women had inspired her upcoming film *9 to 5*, a comedy about corporate secretaries gone rogue. She would produce the film and costar in it, alongside Dolly Parton and Lily Tomlin. She told audiences, "My movie's gonna be a feminist revenge fantasy." They would erupt in cheers.

From the moment the doors to the Workout swung open, the studio was a sensation. Women from across Los Angeles—and in time, tourists from across the country and world—filled the classes and packed the classrooms. "It was like an avalanche," Jane wrote, as the relatively small studio welcomed more than two thousand students daily. Her stepmother, Shirlee, would sometimes work the front desk to keep things running smoothly.

Television crews and popular talk-show hosts like Merv Griffin and Barbara Walters showed up to film Jane in her new role as exercise guru. They found her decked out in leotard, tights, and leg warmers, instructing women in classrooms that became steamy from the body heat. "Does it burn?" she would yell out. "Because if it doesn't burn, you aren't doing it right!" Jane was surprised and thrilled by the success—though she felt a pang of guilt when she thought about how Jane and Leni's Workout had become Jane Fonda's Workout.

The trouble started when Jane began to work with a lawyer to discuss how, exactly, the business should be structured. The lawyer explained that, from a tax perspective, CED should own the business outright. But if Leni wasn't an owner, what would her role be, exactly? "No one, least of all me, ever imagined that the Workout could become as successful as it did. So round and round we went, me with the lawyer," Jane wrote. "What to do about Leni?"

In her memoir, Jane says retelling this story is painful. "Looking back, I see so clearly that the answer to 'What to do about Leni?' was to talk to her, find out what she wanted and what it would take to make us both feel that our needs were addressed," she continued. "Instead I let the lawyer frame the debate, putting Leni into the position of adversary who (we were sure) would fight against CED owning the business."

What would Leni have told Jane, if she had asked?

Leni wanted to retain at least some ownership of the workout she had created—and earn enough money to support herself and her daughter. Instead, Jane's lawyer presented her with a "crappy, crappy contract." She would essentially be just an instructor again. "After the studio was built and was ready to open up, it just turned into something else," Leni told me. "It wasn't mine anymore."

Beyond Leni's original workout, Jane also hired instructors to teach ballet, jazz, funk, and stretch classes.

Meanwhile, Leni had started dating a wealthy land developer who was also an avid sailor. They planned to marry, and with her career taking a tumble, she decided she would take off for a two-year voyage around the world on a sailboat called *Free Spirit*. Leni bowed out of her partnership with Jane graciously, telling her that life was calling her to sea. She even passed along the name of a fellow Gilda Marx instructor and friend who could help Jane manage the studio day-to-day. Her relationship with Jane had begun with an homage to the open waters, and it would end that way—for now.

From nearly the beginning, Jane Fonda's Workout pitched itself as offering women more than a brush with a movie star and a good sweat. An early promotional brochure for the studio reads like a direct predecessor of the contemporary culture of self-care. "The Workout represents a holistic approach to physical and mental wellness," the brochure promised, and aimed "to fulfill people's physical [and] emotional needs." It continues: "There are days when the deep-working discipline of ballet or slow stretch is exactly what you want. Other days you'll want the challenges of a fast-paced workout or jazz class."

Jane assembled a superstar staff to carry out this vision.

There was Jeanne Ernst, the woman Leni recommended. In the late seventies, Jeanne and her husband, a bodybuilder and chiropractor named Bernie Ernst, starred on a fitness TV series called *Body Buddies*. TV executives saw potential in the couple after they appeared on a local talk show with bodybuilding hotshot Arnold Schwarzenegger and Jeanne had the gumption to "call out" Schwarzenegger when he claimed he didn't take vitamins. (Jeanne knew he did.)

Hey, you've got spunk! they told her.

When *The Jack LaLanne Show* went off the air after a quarter of a century, *Body Buddies* replaced it. While Bernie would offer health and weightlifting instruction, Jeanne—usually dressed in a sparkly leotard, tights, and high heels—would lead viewers through a disco dance exercise routine and demonstrate to women how to lift weights. ("No women were lifting weights in those days.") The couple released a *Body Buddies* book, too, and appeared in commercials and infomercials for fitness and weight-loss gadgets.

Shortly after the Workout launched, Jane Fonda hired her to help manage the studio, and—at Jeanne's suggestion—teach a beginner version of what had been Leni's workout. ("People were walking out of that advanced class dying!" Jeanne told me in an interview.)

There was also Doreen Rivera, who was hired to teach funk and stretch classes. Doreen grew up in a Puerto Rican family who was always dancing, and she dreamed of someday dancing professionally. After marrying young and having two daughters, she went on to perform at nightclubs before replacing dancer Toni Basil (later of "Mickey" fame) in one of the country's first breakdancing troupes, called the Lockers.

Then there was Janice Darling, one of the few Black fitness instructors of the era. Janice had always loved to push her body to the limits of its physical potential. As a little girl, she idolized Jack LaLanne and wowed at her school talent show by jumping rope with impossible speed. But when a high school coach recruited her to run track, her father forbade it. Sweat, muscle, competition—none of it was becoming on a young woman, he believed. Particularly not on a Black woman.

In her twenties, while studying acting and dance in Los Angeles, Janice got a job working as a fitness instructor at one of Jack LaLanne's eponymous health spas. When she learned that Jane Fonda was opening a studio nearby, she couldn't resist the opportunity to meet the actress. Who knows, she thought, maybe she could even land an audition for *9 to 5*. Jane didn't cast her in the film, but she did hire her to teach the advanced version of the Workout.

Janice's popularity grew when she began to encourage mental as well as physical strength in class after surviving a horrific accident.

One night after class while waiting in line for a movie, Janice was hit by a car that jumped the curb. The force sent her through a glass storefront, crushing her pelvis, breaking both of her legs, and severing her left eye muscle. She would later credit her fitness routine with helping her to recover. "Being in good shape is not just looking good," she said. "My muscles were so toned and so strong they literally saved my life!" When we spoke for this book, she put it this way: "Every time I taught classes, it wasn't just about the lunges or the leg lifts or the ab work. It was about, all right, let's take that and now let's rise. Let's get the best from ourselves."

Who were the thousands of clients who passed through the doors of the Workout daily? The studio attracted Hollywood hotshots and celebrities, secretaries and housewives. Stars including Ali MacGraw and *Gilligan's Island*'s Tina Louise were regulars; even Ronald Reagan's daughter, Patti Davis, showed up. But so did noncelebrity women who could afford the $5.50 price of admission, or about $17.60 today—a rate that, critics pointed out, meant the studio wasn't quite the democratic haven Jane might have wanted it to be. A few men showed up, too. Some were interested in working out, others saw the studio as a prime pickup spot. (Jeanne Ernst remembers several romances sprouting from her classes.)

The former Jane Fonda Workout studio regulars I interviewed for this book remember the space as having no frills—each classroom was equipped with a simple wood floor, mirrored walls, windows, and a ballet barre. The air-conditioning would sometimes break down in the summer, and with up to fifty people in a class, the mirrors would often become completely fogged over. It had a small changing area and bathroom.

Once classes started, the vibe was intense. Most of the clients were young—no one remembered anyone over fifty in class—and nearly all were trim. For some women, the studio was a rejuvenating and exciting escape; for others, it felt competitive and occasionally catty, as women jockeyed for spots in front of the mirror.

When *Los Angeles Times* writer Pearl Rowe visited the Workout in January 1980, she was struck by how impossibly fit and coordinated the so-called regular women at the studio seemed to be. "[They] gave me the feeling that I'd slipped through a time warp or maybe dozed off during the freezing over of Hell," she wrote. "I walked down the hall and looked in a large window. There was a disco class going on that looked like the Rockettes '79. Their wanton movements to the hellcat music were good enough to sell tickets."

Over the next few years, Jane and Jeanne opened Workout studios in Encino and San Francisco. Together, the studios brought in roughly $20,000 a month in profits—every dime of which went to Tom's political career and CED. While Jane didn't hide the fact that the business existed to fund progressive politics—she spoke frankly about it in interviews—staff and clients didn't spend much time thinking about this connection. "We were there to do fitness," Jeanne told me. "We exercised and we ran the business, and that was it."

———————

The Workout's phenomenal success soon led to a splashy publishing deal with Simon & Schuster. The book that followed would bring her regimen into homes far and wide, spreading her fitness philosophy around the globe.

At Simon & Schuster, Jane worked with famed book editor Nan Talese. It was a fortuitous collaboration: Talese, a client of the Lotte Berk Method studio in New York and the editor of Lydia Bach's *Awake! Aware! Alive!*, understood the power of what Jane was selling. The women "got along wonderfully because I love exercise too," she told a reporter in 1990.*

While working on the book, Talese flew to L.A. to visit the Workout studio. "Jane wanted to know whether I could really do all of the exercises," she told me. (Talese, who is married to writer Gay Talese, also remembered, "She was [very] interested in my marriage. She kept asking questions about my marriage.")

To create *Jane Fonda's Workout Book*, amid running a business and filming and protesting, Jane teamed up with a fellow activist and writer named Mignon McCarthy. The finished product is both a testament to how far women had come since the 1950s and a reflection of what was then Jane's limited understanding of feminism. "Like a great many women, I am a product of a culture that says thin is better, blond is beautiful, and buxom is best," she writes in the book's prologue. "I internalized this message and, in an effort to conform

———————

* Around the same time, Talese would also start working with another uber famous feminist, the dystopian novelist Margaret Atwood, noting: "It seemed to me that she was writing about my life." Women contain multitudes.

to the sought-after female image I abused my health, starved my body, and ingested heaven-knows-what chemical drugs." She decided to write the book, she says, "not because I consider myself an expert in the pedigreed sense, but because I want to share what I've had to learn the hard way with other women."

Jane encourages women to "break the 'weaker sex' mold" and start thinking of themselves as athletes. "Please remember that your goal is not to get pencil thin or to look like someone else," she writes. "Your goal should be to take your body and make it as healthy, strong, flexible, and well-proportioned as you can."

But she also advised women to approach exercise with the same discipline that she found so liberating: Exercise should be fun, but it should also, well, *burn*. "There are no short cuts," she writes. She has a "frantically busy schedule," but she still manages to make time for fitness. The subtext was clear: If *she* could do it, what's *your* excuse?

Eventually she walks readers through the nitty-gritty of her fitness regimen. Exercises are demonstrated by studio staff—including her stepmother, Shirlee Fonda, and an eye-patched Janice Darling. She also offers a diet guide to "eating for health and beauty" and—in true Jane Fonda fashion—ends with a call to action for environmental justice.

In nearly the same breath that Jane laments the pressures women feel to be thin, Jane herself is still super thin, and the book features only super thin fitness models. Millions of women would spend decades trying to untangle these mixed messages.

In November 1981, the same month *Jane Fonda's Workout Book* hit shelves, Jane stunned the world yet again with her performance in the acclaimed film *On Golden Pond*. Jane plays Chelsea, the daughter of Henry Fonda's character, Norman, in a setup that closely imitated their real-life relationship. Norman and Chelsea's relationship is strained and contentious, and Chelsea finally confronts her dad about the bad blood between them. Jane had taken on the project in hopes of working through their actual tensions by playacting.

But the scene that got people talking was one in which Jane, then forty-three years old, appears in a teeny-tiny bikini before doing a backflip off a dock. "No audience could watch Jane without murmuring in tones of awe, 'Look at that tan!' 'Look at that tone!'" *Time* magazine noted.

Simon & Schuster couldn't have dreamt up better publicity for the book. *Workout* soared to the top of the *New York Times* bestseller list, where it held the number one slot for twenty-one weeks. It was translated into fifty languages.

When the book sold 2 million copies in hardcover, Simon & Schuster "threw Jane a champagne party in their conference room and presented her with a $1.2 million royalty check," wrote Bosworth—the biggest royalty check the publisher had ever written.

Over the next few years, Jane churned out several more bestselling books, including a pregnancy fitness book and a book for navigating menopause, reaching women in nearly every life stage. Her influence on fitness would have been vast if she had stopped there. But the wife of a home video maker had an inspired idea.

———————

When Jane got started in the fitness industry, no one she knew owned a videocassette recorder, more commonly known as a VCR. The device had made its American debut in 1977 at the annual Consumer Electronics Show in Las Vegas, but for most people, it was prohibitively expensive. It cost around $1,280, the equivalent today of roughly $5,000.

Then you actually had to buy something to watch. Want your very own copy of *Star Wars*? When the film was released on VHS cassette in 1982, it cost $120. (That's around $500 today.)

Throughout the early eighties, VCRs gradually dropped in price and found a market. Video stores opened to supply early adopters with home entertainment. But few people were willing to actually buy VHS tapes when they could rent them for a fraction of the cost. And besides, who needed to rewatch a film that many times? (The one entertainment category that saw halfway decent VHS sales was pornography.)

But a Southern California entrepreneur named Stuart Karl had a vision.

After dropping out of college in the early 1970s, the "blond-haired, perpetually smiling California surfer" became a waterbed salesman and quickly discovered that retailers could benefit from a magazine about the business. "When that publication became a modest success, he expanded by buying or starting others, including Spa & Sauna and, as the video cassette craze started, Video Store magazine," *The New York Times* reported in 1988. The more he learned about the video business, the more "Mr. Karl was struck by the near-total emphasis on movie tapes and what he considered a huge unmet demand for non-entertainment cassettes."

In 1980, at twenty-seven, he started Karl Home Video to make cassettes that, he liked to say, "filled the gap between *Jaws* and *Deep Throat*." His roster included tapes on home improvement, CPR instruction, and other niche topics.

The following year, during a trip to New York City, Karl and his wife, Debbie, passed a bookstore with a display of *Jane Fonda's Workout Book* in the window. Debbie had read the book and enjoyed doing its exercises at home. She told her husband: This should be a video!

Stuart loved the idea, and he approached Jane.

She said no.

Jane had already signed on to turn the book into a record album that women could play in their living rooms. "When I got the call I remember thinking, *Home video? What's that?*" Jane wrote. "No one I knew had ever bought a videotape."

Plus, she thought it would be weird for an Oscar-winning actress to appear in such a niche kind of production. "I'm an actor," she thought. "It would look foolish for me to be exercising on-camera."

But Karl kept persisting, and eventually she gave in. They could produce it relatively quickly, she reasoned, and hey, maybe it would bring in some extra money for CED.

Jane hired her friend Sidney Galanty to direct and produce. Galanty had a long history making leftist political ads. He had worked for the Kennedy administration and for Hubert Humphrey's campaign for president. Most recently, he'd worked for CED, making TV ads for Tom Hayden's 1982 run for the California state assembly.

Galanty was up for a change of scenery and a challenge.

Jane wanted the video to feel like a real-life class. For the set, they re-created a studio classroom, complete with a bulletin board and folding chairs around the perimeter. (They would have filmed in Jane's actual studio, but the mirrors were a problem.) She enlisted her favorite instructors to work out behind her.

To save on production costs, Jane told Galanty she wanted everyone to do their own hair and makeup. She wrote a rough script in pencil, sitting on the floor of a hotel room, but she didn't want to use teleprompters. She wanted to try to wing it.

Still, she worried about whether she could carry a ninety-minute video as Jane Fonda, without playing a role. "She'd never done video and was apprehensive," Galanty told *Billboard* in 1985. "And frankly, no one knew if she'd be charismatic and able to reach through that camera and involve the people at home."

The video opens with a close-up of Doreen Rivera stretching at a ballet barre. As the camera pans out, we see more women (and two men) warming up. Eventually, Jane enters, wearing her now-iconic striped pink leotard, belt, pink tights, and leg warmers. The camera settles on a Black woman and a white woman who sit down on the floor and, together, form a *W* with their bodies—it became the

Workout's emblem. Then Jane makes her way to the front of the room and asks, "Are you ready to do the Workout?"

For the next ninety minutes, she leads viewers through her classic exercise routine to upbeat instrumental music. She tells them to "go for the burn" as she bends, bounces, and stretches. Doreen Rivera occasionally whoops in encouragement in the background.

In order to capture this one "class," Jane and her instructors spent three marathon days on set. Every time Galanty needed a new take—maybe someone went left when they should have gone right—Jane and her instructors had to reshoot an entire twenty-five-minute segment. By the end, their bodies had not only gotten a Workout; they had taken a beating. But Galanty knew they had created something special. Jane, he told *Billboard*, "was magic."

Jane Fonda's Workout video would come to influence far more than fitness—the tape is now credited with launching the entire home entertainment industry. "The crucial thing about creating a successful business, I have subsequently realized, is timing—giving people something they really want that they can't yet get anywhere else," Jane wrote. "But at the time I was not aware of how serendipitous our timing was, or that there was a budding video industry poised to explode."

At first *Jane Fonda's Workout* video sales were slow. When the tape appeared in stores in May 1982, it sold for a retail price of $59.95—the equivalent of $159 today—and moved only 3,000 copies its first month. But as Jane relentlessly promoted the video, just as she had her bestselling book before it, and word of mouth spread, "we could sense the groundswell," Stuart Karl told *Billboard*. "The tape began to gain a very steady momentum."

In order to benefit from the Workout, Jane told fans they had to do it regularly, which meant they had to own a copy. The tape was pricey, but for the many women who didn't have the time or income to take exercise classes at a studio—as well as for those who felt more comfortable sweating in the privacy of their living room—the cassette was a gift.

Before long, *Jane Fonda's Workout* rocketed to number four on *Billboard*'s videocassette sales chart, and it soon worked its way up to number one, where it remained for forty-one weeks. Until then, the most successful home videos sold around 25,000 copies; *Workout* sold more than 200,000 in its first year alone. It would go on to sell 17 million copies, becoming one of the bestselling home videos of all time.

From there, Jane churned out one video after another with Stuart Karl and Sid Galanty. There was a video for more advanced students and one for beginners; there was *Jane Fonda's Pregnancy, Birth and Recovery Workout* and *Jane Fonda's New Workout*. They all sold like gangbusters.

Gradually Jane moved away from telling her acolytes to "go for the burn." The newly formed IDEA Health and Fitness, the first national organization for fitness professionals, launched in 1982, and its leadership had discovered that high-impact aerobics were causing widespread injuries, including stress fractures and back problems, among devotees. Medical experts had concerns as well. For her *New Workout*, Jane began working with Dr. James G. Garrick, an orthopedic surgeon and then director of San Francisco's Center for Sports Medicine, to create a safer, lower-impact program.

She also reached out to Dr. Ken Cooper, the father of aerobics, after he commented during a TV interview that he didn't support "going for the burn." The problem, he said, was potential confusion among ambitious exercisers over where that burn was supposed to be happening. Burning in the thighs was one thing; burning in the chest was another. He told the interviewer he advised against exercising to the point of pain or extreme discomfort. "That could be something that you want to avoid, even something for which you need to seek medical consultation."

Not long after the interview, Cooper received a letter in the mail from Jane. When he saw her name on the envelope, he thought, *Oh boy, lawsuit.* To the contrary, he told me, Jane was writing to seek his advice. "Dr. Cooper, you've been in the business a whole lot longer than me," Cooper remembers her writing. "You've made mistakes, and I've made my mistakes. Why don't we work together and see if we can make it safe for most people?"

Cooper appreciated Jane's eagerness to learn and was glad to offer his guidance. For a while, his fitness and cardiovascular institute in Dallas reviewed Jane's videos before they were released. "Jane Fonda was smart enough to realize that this could be a passing fad, that it could be dangerous," he told me, if she didn't ground what she was advocating in actual science.

Jane was forever adapting, said Jeanne Ernst. She would say: "You do the best with what you've got at the moment, and when you find out how to do it differently, you do."

By the mid-eighties, Jane and the larger dance aerobics universe had also begun wearing a hot new accessory: shoes. Throughout the seventies and early eighties, most aerobics instructors and students exercised barefoot. (Jacki Sorensen and her devotees were a notable exception to this trend.) When they did wear sneakers, "they were appropriated from other sports," writes journalist Nicholas Smith in *Kicks: The Great American Story of Sneakers.* Over time, the lack of appropriate footwear took a toll on aerobicizers' feet and legs.

Nike might have seemed the obvious choice to pounce on the aerobics market. The shoe company had grown from a tiny upstart at the beginning of the seventies into a juggernaut by riding the jogging wave. But Nike founder Phil Knight showed little interest in capitalizing on women's exercise culture. "Nike was working hard to ignore the fitness boom," writes Smith, much to the frustration of women in the company who recognized its potential. This left the market wide open for another player to seize the opportunity.

The British shoe brand Reebok danced onto the stage.

Angel Martinez, a West Coast sales rep for Reebok, first dreamt up an aerobics shoe when he stopped by his wife's exercise class and heard women complaining of aches and pains. After a few failed attempts, he sold Reebok executives on the idea, and they ordered up a prototype from their manufacturer in East Asia.

"Martinez took the prototype to fitness instructors, who loved it," writes Smith. The shoe had come back from the factory with a wrinkle around the toe, which the factory owner apologized for but Reebok executives liked. It made the shoe resemble a ballet slipper.

They told the factory to keep the wrinkles in.

In 1982, Reebok officially debuted its Freestyle fitness sneaker in white, pastel pink, and pastel blue. "The upper was made of garment or glove leather, much softer and more pliable than the leather used for other sneakers at the time," writes Smith. "Freestyle wearers found them so comfortable that they didn't need to be broken in."

Early on, Reebok gave out free pairs of Freestyles to aerobics instructors across the country, whose students then rushed to buy pairs of their own. And as workout wear spilled over from the studio to the street, women bought them as everyday shoes, too.

"The Freestyle rocketed Reebok's sales from $1.5 million the year before the shoe hit the market to nearly $13 million the year after," notes Smith. By 1987, Reebok had soared past Nike in domestic shoe sales, as the Freestyle became the shoe of the decade.

The *Workout* books and tapes propelled Jane from celebrity to idol. Around the globe, women were "doing Jane," as her fans cutely called her regimen, by the millions. Exercisers worshiped her for her beauty and vigor, her perceived credibility and authenticity. By 1984, the *World Almanac* ranked Jane the fourth most influential woman in the world, behind Mother Teresa, Margaret Thatcher, and Nancy Reagan.

Jane began to receive a deluge of letters—"touching, handwritten letters" that she saved. "These women poured their hearts out, about weight they had lost, self-esteem they had gained, how they were finally able to stand up to their boss or recover from a mastectomy, asthma, respiratory failure, diabetes," she wrote. "One woman described how, brushing her teeth one morning, she was stunned to see arm muscles in the mirror for the first time."

A Peace Corps volunteer told Jane she exercised to an audiocassette version of the Workout in a mud hut in Guatemala. A woman I interviewed for this book whose husband was in the foreign service recounted "doing Jane" in Cairo, Egypt.

Jane discovered that women now felt a new kind of intimacy toward her. "When your voice and image are coming into someone's living room (or mud hut) every day . . . you become part of people's lives in a personal way, different from movie stars on the big screen," she wrote. "They felt they knew me."

At times, she worried the Workout was subsuming everything else about her. "What about me as an actor? What about the causes I am fighting for?" she wrote. "I didn't want pelvic tilts to define me." But she also found herself becoming increasingly invested in the business. "I wanted to see it make a difference—not just for wealthy women in Beverly Hills."

For millions, it did. But for many, Jane's brand of fitness brought mixed feelings, as the joy of the early years of dance aerobics became co-opted by a cultural mandate that women strive for physical perfection. As aerobics pioneer Debbie Rosas told researcher Beth Swanson: While aerobic dancing began as "a very feminine impulse," over time, "it absorbed a male attitude." Some argued it became a tool of the patriarchy. More and more, aerobics was pitched as a path not only to slim down but to strive for a physique biologically unattainable for most—that is to say, Jane Fonda's physique: long, impossibly lean, and muscular. Women exerted themselves, but it wasn't always in the service of strength. By the end of the decade, many feminists would argue that the rise of Jane Fonda was not a triumph of feminism but a backlash to it.

In the early eighties, the first wave of baby boomers—the generation that defined and created "youth culture"—were nearing forty. But they had no intention of growing old in the same way their parents had. And increasingly, culture and capitalism told them they didn't have to. After all, even President Reagan was attempting to turn back the clock on his physique.

Advertising agencies began to sell the idea aging was not in fact inevitable, if you bought the right face cream or bubble bath. They highlighted the role of "science" in helping personal care companies develop "miracle" antiaging products; for the generation that had watched in awe as man walked on the moon for the first time, this seemed plausible.

At the same time, advertisers began to push the idea that for the modern woman, "empowerment" essentially meant spending money on oneself. "By the 1980s, advertising agencies had figured out how to make feminism—and antifeminism—work for them," wrote Susan J. Douglas in *Where the Girls Are*. "Women's liberation became equated with women's ability to do whatever they wanted for themselves, whenever they wanted, no matter what the expense."

In short: They had figured out how to commodify feminism.

If there was one emblematic ad campaign of the 1980s, Douglas writes, it was actress Cybill Shepherd hawking Preference by L'Oréal hair coloring with the slogan "I'm worth it." That slogan became a kind of motto for women during the decade, she wrote. "In stark contrast to the selfless wife and mom of *The Feminine Mystique*, not to mention those hideous, loudmouthed feminists who thought sisterhood and political activism mattered, women of the 1980s were urged to take care of themselves, and to do so *for* themselves."

In Jane, women found a path both to feminism and becoming more conventionally beautiful in a culture that still valued women for their appearance above everything else. Here was an incredibly impressive woman—an Oscar-winning filmmaker and actor, a world-changing activist—whose role as a mother and devoted wife made her uniquely accessible to Middle America. Not only that, she was in her *forties*, with the body and energy of a much younger woman.

Why *not* follow her lead?

———————

Among many Workout colleagues, Jane was revered. She engaged with her staff and made herself as accessible as possible. "She drove her own car," Julie Lafond (who was hired by Jane to be the CEO of Workout enterprises in 1984) told me—a beat-up Volvo station wagon. "She did her own shopping. I mean, she tried to live as normal a life as she possibly could."

Gerry Puhara, the costume director for several of her videos in the 1980s, agreed: "When it was time to have lunch, she'd sit with everybody and chat. She was very open, and she'd discuss her life. And of course, everyone really adored her, was in awe of her."

Well, not everyone. Throughout the eighties, Jane faced a series of multimillion-dollar lawsuits by staff that called her apparent beliefs in equality and empowerment into question. In 1983, three women who had been instructors at her San Francisco Workout studio filed a $3 million lawsuit for sex discrimination after they discovered male instructors were paid more per hour. In *The New York Times*, Jane's lawyer is quoted as calling the suit "frivolous and totally without merit," because "The male who was receiving $8.50 an hour was a head trainer."

In 1987, a former Beverly Hills Workout instructor named

Audrey Pressman filed a $2.3 million suit, alleging Jane and the company conspired to steal her clients. "The lawsuit claims the Workout induced Ms. Pressman's clients to buy yearlong memberships with promises she would continue to be an instructor. However, she claims the defendants were actually planning to fire her," the Associated Press reported.

For a while, Gilda Marx considered suing Jane, too—for "ripping her off" by offering classes that were strikingly similar to the ones taught at her studio. But when she consulted with a lawyer, she had to admit that Jane's success hadn't actually hurt her business; to the contrary, it had fueled it. In the end, she told me in an interview, "Jane actually helped me. [Her success] turned out to be very positive for the whole industry."

Jane began to realize that the Workout was changing her. It changed her perception of herself. She began to feel truly strong for the first time in her life. "There was something about taking control of my body in that way," she said. "I know now that, for me, the moving to the music, the endorphins, the sweating, led me into the long, slow process of accepting my own body."

The process would take decades. "I had stopped bingeing and purging, but I wasn't really healed," she wrote. "I was the way a dry drunk is in relationship to alcohol." When it came to exercise, she later said, she was "way too compulsive." But the strength she was drawing from the Workout would continue to deepen. It would also help her "remain intact during the dark times that lay ahead."

The irony of the Workout as a tool for women's empowerment was, of course, that it existed to fund her husband's ambition. It was all for Tom—who, it just so happened, couldn't stand Jane's new career.

In 1982, the Workout's success got Tom elected to the California state assembly—his first public office. "Hayden's campaign had been the most expensive state legislature campaign in U.S. history," wrote Bosworth. The Workout's profits, combined with Jane's glamour and devotion, "had made the victory possible, more so than Hayden's 'Growing Up with America' slogan and his new moderate positions."

Still, Tom thought the Workout was "an exercise in vanity."

"Tom hated, loathed, despised the Workout," Jane's stepdaughter Nathalie Vadim told Bosworth. "Now Jane was not only a movie star; she was a one-woman conglomerate, a veritable household word—an icon." And Tom, she continued, "could not take it. The Workout overwhelmed his politics, his sense of self, as well as everything in their life together."

Tom had started to drink heavily and have affairs. For a while, Jane turned a blind eye. She worshiped Tom and believed he gave her credibility as an activist. "Tom's the intelligent one; I'm just a chameleon," she would say. When she was around him, she would defer to him entirely. "She lived with a duality: outspoken, creative, independent lady versus victimized, inferior little girl," wrote Bosworth. "Such extremes! But she played both roles to a fare-thee-well."

In 1986, Jane and Julie Lafond decided to split the Workout from CED and transfer ownership to Jane. It was purely a business decision, Julie told me, meant to fuel the Workout's growth. In all, the fitness business had brought in $17 million for CED. "I felt we had more than fulfilled our original mission of providing it with a solid financial base," Jane wrote. It was time to move on.

In late 1989, after seventeen years of marriage, Jane and Tom also decided to split. The divorce was immeasurably painful for Jane. But at fifty-two years old, she was one step closer to being able to define her life on her own terms.

Jane would go through several more "acts," as she has called each circumscribed stage of her life. In 1991, she closed the original Workout studio. "An era in exercise has ended," wrote the *Los Angeles Times*, "the aerobics studio that launched a multimillion-dollar fitness empire took a permanent breather." While the studio had continued to be profitable, it struggled to compete with the influx of new health clubs "offering everything from juice bars to racquet-ball."

That same year, she married CNN founder, rancher, and billion-aire Ted Turner, who had pursued her as soon as the news of her split from Tom became public. Jane moved to Atlanta, where Ted was based, and (temporarily) retired from acting to become a full-time wife and philanthropist.

The decade-plus that Jane spent in Atlanta—the first time she had lived in a city other than New York or L.A. or Paris—was en-lightening. "She found out about real people," Julie Lafond told me. "It was different from Hollywood. As much as she had tried to be out among the real people before, that's hard to do in Hollywood." (When I was growing up in Atlanta, the city embraced Jane as a hometown hero; there weren't a lot of celebrities cruising down Peachtree Street in those days. She became a fixture at Braves base-ball games and local hot spots.)

Jane's daughter, Vanessa Vadim, also moved to Atlanta, along with a daughter she and Tom had adopted, Mary Luana "Lulu" Wil-liams. During this time, Jane became a grandmother. "No one had prepared me for the feelings that arose when I held this little boy, Vanessa's child," she wrote. "I was utterly broken open in ways I had never been before. Malcolm had enabled me to discover the combina-tion to the safe where the soft spot of my heart had been shut away for so long."

In 2001, Jane and Ted divorced, after she found herself feeling stifled in their marriage. Eventually she returned to Hollywood—and to acting and activism.

Jane also reunited with Leni Cazden, her original partner in those early days of Jane and Leni's Workout, who had been watching

Jane's life unfurl from a (short) distance. In the original *Jane Fonda Workout Book*'s acknowledgments, Jane thanks Leni, "wherever you are."

In fact, Leni was a mile away in Santa Monica, hoping for the day when Jane would acknowledge her in a more official way.

In a strange turn of events, many years after they parted ways, when Jane was married to Ted Turner, Leni began working as Ted's fitness trainer at an ultra-exclusive gym in Los Angeles, where he spent time on business. Leni had long since given up teaching exercise classes—when she returned to L.A. after sailing around the world, the group fitness scene had exploded to such a degree she no longer felt special doing what she did. But she came to love working out with weights.

Through her work with Ted, Leni reconnected with Jane. The women even became friends. It was only then that Jane learned about Leni's painful past and began to understand the hurt she had inflicted on her by cutting her out of the Workout.

Jane described this realization in her memoir: "Leni had been robbed of the ability to speak up on her own behalf," she wrote. "The word *no* was not part of her vocabulary, and she had felt powerless earlier to negotiate with me and the lawyer. Had we been able to sit face-to-face as women—Leni owning her voice and me not ceding mine to the lawyer—things could have been worked out."

After Leni was able to express her hurt and anger, Jane also compensated her financially, offering her "enough to live comfortably." But it wasn't until October 2020—as I was finishing writing this chapter—that Jane and Leni appeared *together* in an interview for the first time, to share their story with the world and for Jane to make things right. The Slate podcast *Decoder Ring*, hosted by television critic Willa Paskin, featured the women in a two-part episode on the origins and triumph of the Workout video, and Leni finally got the credit she felt she deserved. "If I were then where I am now—in my head and my heart—it would have gone down differently," Jane tells Leni. She had felt guilty about what happened for forty years. Leni responds: "We can let that go now."

Leni also shared, as she had told me a few months prior, that despite what life had dealt her, she was doing just fine. "It's nuts that I should end up happy," she says. "And yet, I really am."

In the years after leaving Ted, Jane finally began to fully confront her two lifelong demons: existing to please men and doing so by attempting to be perfect. After spending so much of her life fearing that if she *wasn't* perfect she wouldn't be loved, she began to realize that "wanting to be perfect is to want the impossible."

In her memoir, she explains, "Perfect is for God: Completion, as Carl Jung said, is what we humans should strive for. But completion (wholeness) isn't possible until we stop trying to be perfect. The tyranny of perfection forced me to confuse spiritual hunger with physical hunger." She then adds: "This toxic striving for perfection is a female thing. How many men obsess about being perfect? For men, generally, good enough is good enough."

Jane's feminist breakthrough came during a performance of Eve Ensler's *The Vagina Monologues*. She wrote: "I had no idea what to expect, but as I sat there listening to Eve enact the monologues she'd written based on interviews she'd done with women about their vaginas, I felt something happening to me. I don't remember ever laughing so hard or crying so hard in the theater, but it must have been during the laughter part, when I wasn't paying attention, that my feminist consciousness slipped out of my head and took up residence in my body—where it has lived ever since."

This doesn't mean Jane has stopped caring about her appearance. "I'm glad that I look good for my age, but I've also had plastic surgery. I'm not going to lie about that," she said in 2018. "On one level, I hate the fact that I have had the need to alter myself physically to feel that I'm OK. I wish that I wasn't like that. . . . I wish I was braver, but I am what I am."

———————

In the years after Jane's original Workout book and video hit shelves, the country saw a deluge of imitators. Fitness-minded celebrities watched Jane's success and believed they, too, could inspire women to move—or at least to spend money on the particular brand of fitness they were selling. In 1983, *Dallas* star Victoria Principal published *The Body Principal*, which replaced Jane's *Workout* as number one on the *New York Times* bestseller list. The following year, actress Raquel Welch released her *Total Beauty and Fitness* video, which in deliciously gaudy fashion married the decade's obsession with fitness and luxury. It begins with shots of Welch on the deck of a private boat; then she emerges from the ocean in a zebra-striped bathing suit and sparkling earrings, before moving through a well-appointed patio to her workout stage, reinforcing the message that a fit body is an *expensive* body.

Debbie Reynolds, an icon of Old Hollywood, got in on the game, too, producing one of the most remarkably kitschy artifacts from the early eighties fitness explosion. The *Singin' in the Rain* star's 1983 video, *Do It Debbie's Way*, featured the then-fifty-one-year-old actress leading a calisthenics-style workout meant to be a gentler alternative to Jane's feel-the-burn approach—a chance to "fun around" while breaking a sweat. The video includes some of Reynolds's celebrity friends as backup exercisers, including Dionne Warwick, Teri Garr, Florence Henderson, and a stoic Shelley Winters, dressed in a black sweatshirt that reads "I'm only doing this for Debbie." The women move against a lush backdrop of pink curtains and pink carpet, Debbie's name in floor-to-ceiling lights, as they bend and stretch to swing classics like "In the Mood." Debbie also launched a short-lived exercise clothing line for "the fuller-figured woman."

Also in 1983, the trailblazing Black model, actress, and broadcaster Jayne Kennedy released a workout video called *Love Your Body*, following the success of her LP and cassette by the same name. Jayne had been crowned Miss Ohio in 1970—the first Black woman to earn the title—and she was the first Black woman to become a sportscaster for a national network, when CBS hired her for *The NFL Today*. She decided to shoot the exercise video after divorcing her first husband, who as her manager had tried to control her career and life. Many of the video's backup exercisers were also people of color.

"I want every one of you out there to love your body," Jayne says in the video's introduction. "Now, when I say, 'Love your body,' I mean that I want you to be healthy, happy, and in shape. Eat right, exercise regularly, and learn what your body needs and love it for what it is. Establish a positive belief in yourself. That's what my exercise program will help you to achieve."

Jayne was one of the only faces of color on fitness video shelves for many years, and she inspired untold numbers of Black women to exercise along with her. The video became a bestseller and sent the message loud and clear: Black women deserved to "love their body," too.

In time, America would also see workouts from Cher and Heather Locklear and a teenaged Alyssa Milano. *Murder, She Wrote* star Angela Lansbury released a video for older women. "Marky Mark" Wahlberg made a fitness video, as did I Can't Believe It's Not Butter! spokesman Fabio, whose exercise cues are punctuated with dramatic tosses of his long blond hair. Some of these stars knew what they were doing; others, not so much.

For home exercisers who wanted to feel confident that they were working out with a true pro, one could choose from among a growing list of videos starring fitness instructors inspired by Jane who became celebrities in their own right. There was Kathy Smith—another early student of Gilda Marx, who had served as one of the

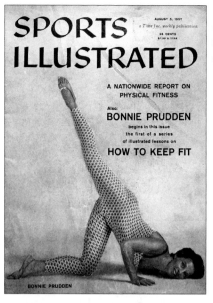

Fitness pioneer Bonnie Prudden graces the cover of *Sports Illustrated*, August 5, 1957.

Prudden demonstrates trampoline exercises at her Institute of Physical Fitness in White Plains, New York, circa 1955.

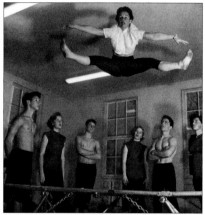

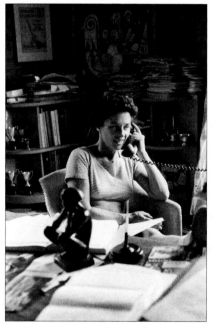

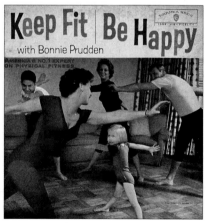

Prudden's *Keep Fit / Be Happy* record, released by Warner Bros. Records in 1960, encouraged Americans to exercise at home—a novel concept at the time.

Prudden gets down to business in her office at the institute, late 1950s.

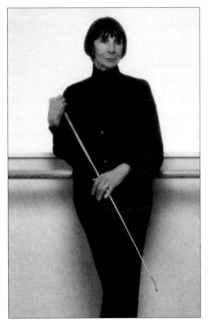

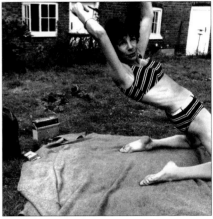

Berk lounges in the garden of her daughter's home in Berkshire, England, early 1960s.

Lotte Berk, creator of the barre workout, with her trademark whip, circa 1981.

Berk with her daughter, Esther Fairfax, early 1960s.

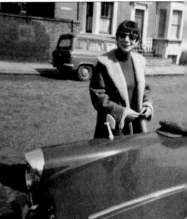

Berk shows off her first sports car, mid-1960s.

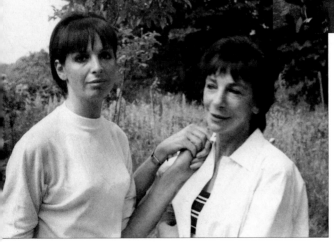

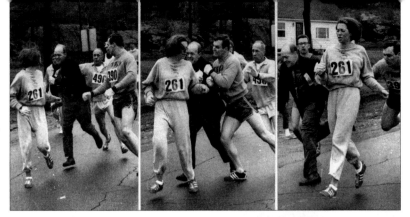

Boston Marathon co-director Jock Semple attempts to forcibly remove Kathrine Switzer from the race, 1967.

Bobbi Gibb barrels toward the finish line of the 1966 Boston Marathon, becoming the first woman to complete the course.

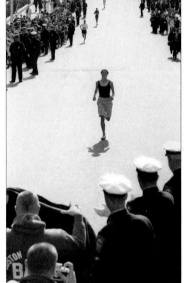

Switzer (*fourth from left*) at the start of New York Road Runners' inaugural Crazylegs Mini-Marathon, the country's first women-only road race, 1972.

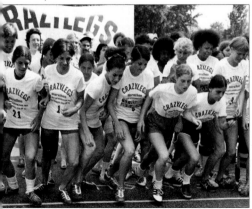

Advertisement for the first modern sports bra, late 1970s.

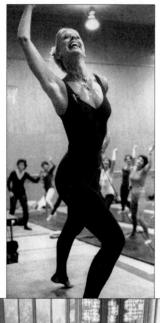

Jazzercise creator Judi Sheppard Missett in her element, 1979.

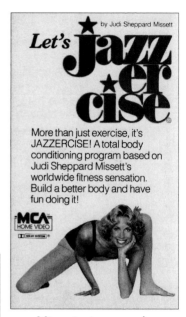

by Judi Sheppard Missett

Let's **Jazzercise**

More than just exercise, it's JAZZERCISE! A total body conditioning program based on Judi Sheppard Missett's worldwide fitness sensation. Build a better body and have fun doing it!

MCA HOME VIDEO

Missett jazzing out on the cover of one of her first home workout cassettes, released by MCA Home Video in 1983.

Flexatard designer Gilda Marx (*center*) at a 1978 fashion show. The model on the far left is budding fitness titan Kathy Smith.

Missett leads a Jazzercise class at the John F. Kennedy Center for the Performing Arts in Washington, D.C., further enshrining the workout as an American institution.

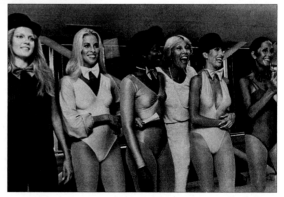

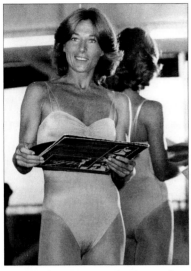

Leni Cazden, the original architect of Jane Fonda's iconic workout, 1978.

Jane Fonda at the opening of her Beverly Hills Workout studio, 1979.

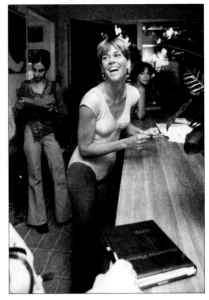

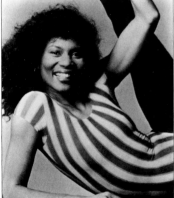

Janice Darling taught at the original Jane Fonda Workout studio in Beverly Hills and posed in *Jane Fonda's Workout Book* before opening her own aerobics studio, the Sweat Shop.

Fonda feels the burn in her chart-topping *Workout* video, 1982.

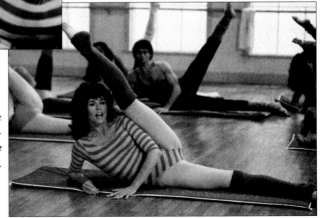

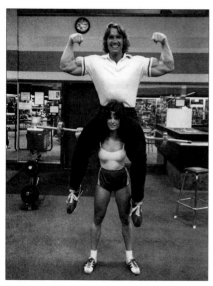

Bodybuilding pioneer Lisa Lyon could deadlift twice her weight—and carry Arnold Schwarzenegger on her shoulders.

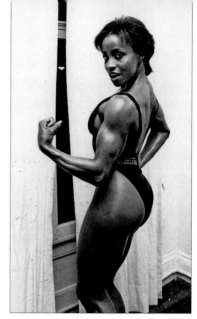

When she was crowned Ms. Olympia in 1983, Carla Dunlap became the first Black woman to win bodybuilding's highest honor.

Time magazine declares strong sexy in this August 30, 1982, cover story.

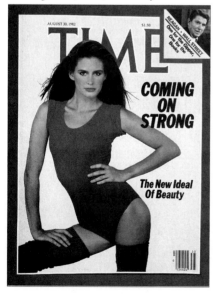

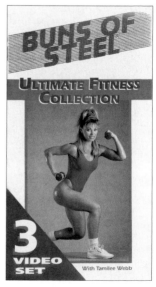

Tamilee Webb flexes on the cover of a *Buns of Steel* home video collection, released by the Maier Group in 1993.

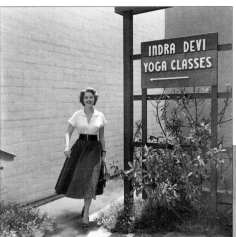

A student visits the Indra Devi Yoga Studio in Hollywood, circa 1952.

Devi instructs the student inside her yoga studio, circa 1952.

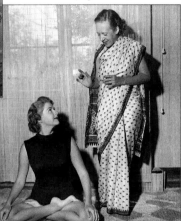

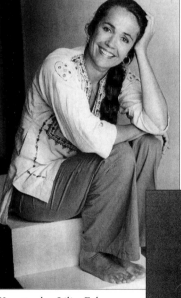

Folan lets loose with Phil Donahue on his daytime talk show, mid-1970s.

Yoga teacher Lilias Folan, host of PBS's *Lilias, Yoga, and You*, in 1976.

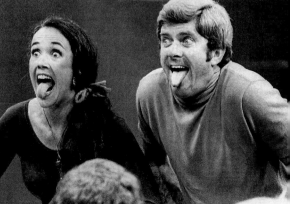

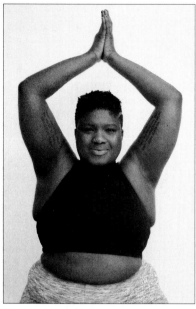

Yoga teacher and Instagram star Jessamyn Stanley is a tireless advocate for body inclusivity in fitness.

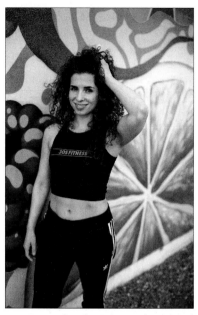

305 Fitness founder Sadie Kurzban created her cardio dance workout to encourage physical pride, not transformation.

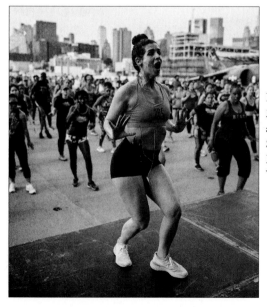

Kurzban instructs a 305 Fitness class aboard the Intrepid Sea, Air & Space Museum in New York City.

first-ever models for the Flexatard. Kathy released her first exercise record and video in the early eighties and built an empire of books and videos from there. In direct competition was Denise Austin, who trained as a gymnast and got her start in the industry as a young demonstrator on *The Jack LaLanne Show*. Jazzercise's Judi Sheppard Missett continued to make videos, too.

By the late eighties, nearly *five hundred* workout videos were being released every year. By then, however, many women began to want more than tone and definition and a good sweat. They wanted nothing less than bodies of steel.

CHAPTER 6

Lift

I have a head for business and a bod for sin.
Is there anything wrong with that?

—Tess McGill, *Working Girl*, 1988

W hen Lisa Lyon slipped into a bikini to compete in the first World Women's Bodybuilding Championship, she hadn't planned to become a crusader for women and muscle. She had just turned twenty-six, and she entered the contest on a lark.

Not that she hadn't trained. For two years she'd pulled back her long dark curls into a ponytail, pulled on a pair of short-shorts, and spent three hours a day, six days a week, weightlifting at the world-famous Gold's Gym in Santa Monica, "the Versailles of the Beefcake Palaces." She was slight, only five-three, but could deadlift 265 pounds—more than twice her bodyweight, if anyone asked. She liked the way her newly muscular body made her feel: like a jaguar, she would tell friends.

Now, in June 1979, she posed on stage alongside nine other

women in downtown Los Angeles's Embassy Auditorium, their biceps and quadriceps glistening with body oil, as a mostly male panel evaluated their muscle definition, symmetry, and overall presentation. Finally the judges of the contest announced their verdict.

Lisa Lyon had won.

Cameras flashed, and with that, she suddenly found herself regarded as a national spokesperson for women's muscle, called on by the press and the public to defend and elucidate a practice most Americans still considered "freakish."

By today's bodybuilding standards (or any standards), Lisa was tiny—a wisp of a woman, at 105 pounds. "Except for her sculptured biceps, she might have been simply a tennis single from the marina or a runner from the beach," observed a writer for *Esquire*. Her competition was small, too. But in the summer of 1979, the fact that these women wanted to flaunt and flex their muscles at all made them newsworthy. "I look at my body in terms of a beautiful, functional female animal," she told a reporter after her win, "a vital, high-technical body which incorporates good health."

Since the fifties, nearly every type of strenuous exercise—jogging and dancing and tucking at a ballet barre—could be spun as a way for women to become lean and lovely. Weightlifting was trickier. Choosing to raise hunks of iron meant seeking out strength for strength's sake, which defied every norm of womanhood. The act itself was rarely graceful, often eliciting grunts and grimaces. Building muscle implied expanding the body, not reducing it. More than any other physical activity, weightlifting, Americans believed, would make women—sin of all sins—look like men.

But in the late seventies, propelled by the spirit of the women's movement and the fitness boom sweeping the country, women became curious: *What did it feel like to pump iron?* Some were encouraged to lift by enlightened boyfriends or husbands. Others wanted to show less enlightened partners they could be strong, too. And still others had always enjoyed testing their physical power but hadn't had access to what were previously the exclusively male spaces of weight rooms and lifting gyms—until now.

In time, the rise of the seriously muscular woman would inspire even casual observers to view women's capacity for strength more expansively. Even Gloria Steinem found herself reconsidering the outer limits of women's potential when she interviewed a champion powerlifter and bodybuilder in the mid-eighties. "Just to give you an idea what an impact meeting one strong woman can have: I went out and bought weights," she wrote in *Moving Beyond Words*. "We're talking personal revolution here. Though I wouldn't want to oversell my progress, it was the beginning of my finding a way out of the fat-versus-thin dichotomy this country presents."

With her win at the World Championship, the first women's bodybuilding contest to be sanctioned by the Amateur Athletic Union, Lisa Lyon was now the most visible of these early adopters. And she turned her experience into a rallying cry.

Weightlifting had transformed Lisa's life. Growing up in Beverly Hills, the daughter of an "orthodontist to the stars" and an interior designer, she was frail and shy. Her shoulders and hips turned inward. She spoke softly and developed what she considered "esoteric" passions—she dreamed of becoming an illustrator for medical textbooks and made a study of human anatomy.

She had trained in dance when she was young, but her first real taste of strength came in college. One night on the campus of UCLA, where she was majoring in anthropology, she encountered a group of male students dressed in cloaks and carrying bamboo swords. She wasn't scared so much as intrigued. "Who *are* you?" she asked.

She learned they practiced a Japanese martial art called kendo, and she asked if she could join their club. They agreed, but told her they wouldn't go easy on her just because she was a girl.

Shortly into her kendo training, Lisa decided she needed to

strengthen her upper body (all the better to wield her bamboo sword). That's when she started lifting. She discovered she liked the way weight training made her feel. She liked it so much, in fact, that she wanted to spend every spare minute pumping iron. There was weightlifting and bench-pressing and deadlifting (gym-speak for raising heavy objects off the ground), complemented by push-ups and pull-ups and running staircases. "Here was something I could create," she told a reporter in late 1979, "building in the most positive sense as opposed to 'slim and trim' or losing weight or avoiding getting fat or all the reasons that women exercise that are negative."

She convinced the management at Gold's Gym to let her train in its bodybuilders' mecca, where the sounds of clinking metal mixed with rock and roll, and she "fell in love with the scene." Her stint with the kendo club had given her practice being the only woman in the room, but it wasn't always easy. "A lot of the men bodybuilders there resented being invaded by a woman," she said at the time. "But after a while they realized that I was serious about bodybuilding, and they became very helpful."

Among those helpful men was the king of bodybuilding himself.

In the late seventies, Arnold Schwarzenegger was an uber-ambitious Austrian expat who had risen to become the sport's biggest star. Handsome and goofily charming with a devilish smile, he had sculpted his body into something resembling a comic book superhero—only much, much bigger. He had just made his dramatic film debut alongside Jeff Bridges and Sally Field in the bodybuilding drama *Stay Hungry*, and he had won bodybuilding's highest honor, the Mr. Olympia title, so many times that by his late twenties, when he met Lisa Lyon, he announced he was retiring.

But Arnold's greatest feat may have been making bodybuilding aspirational. Through force of personality, he almost single-handedly shifted bodybuilding's reputation from being a marginal pastime to a respectable activity for regular middle- and upper-class guys, inspiring them to supplement their jogging and racquetball regimens with rounds of heavy lifting.

The first time Arnold met Lisa—out one night, with a friend—she appeared so "fragile" he worried "if he said the wrong thing she might break down and cry." The next time he saw her, however, he didn't even recognize her. "Instead of the frail girl I met," he told writer Douglas Kent Hall, "Lisa had transformed herself into this incredibly strong woman." Strong, and also sexy. When Arnold saw Lisa guest-pose at a Mr. Los Angeles competition, he was awed. "Look at the latissimus, the rear deltoids!" he exclaimed. *Isn't she fantastic?*

Lisa was equally impressed by Arnold. "When I met Arnold Schwarzenegger, I saw there was potential to do something dramatic with myself," she told *Esquire*'s Eve Babitz, who noted "her perfect little Bardot-Ronstadt face," sparkling brown eyes, and white teeth. Lisa and Arnold began training together. In time, she decided: She wanted to do for women what Arnold had done for men—to expand the definition of feminine beauty to include serious muscle.

When she wasn't coming or going from Gold's Gym, Lisa dressed in leather motorcycle jackets and tight pants. To earn a paycheck, she had a job reading books and scripts for American International Pictures. She had been courted by actor Jack Nicholson as a college student and would soon begin dating the French rock star Bernard Lavilliers. But in the heady few years after her contest win, her heart was in bodybuilding. The International Federation of Bodybuilding asked Lisa to chair a brand-new women's committee and help organize two more women's bodybuilding contests planned for Atlantic City. She became a one-woman public relations machine set on changing Americans' beliefs about women and muscle.

"In every era, the definition of female beauty has a lot to do with the woman's role in society," she told a reporter after her win, drawing on her anthropology degree. "In the 60s, there was the skinny body—beautiful but kind of decadent. I think going into the 80s we need something that will correspond to power."

In time, Lisa's influence would extend beyond the small weight-lifting subculture and into big-box gyms and middle-class living rooms across America, as women with no intention of posing on a stage wanted hard bodies, too. By the end of the decade, the new beauty ideal for American women was a body so firm you could bounce a quarter off it. This was surely progress for women. But it came at a cost.

———————

The birth of women's bodybuilding revealed just how strong women could be when given the chance to train alongside men. But because bodybuilding was, at its core, a beauty contest—a sport whose end goal was aesthetic—it provided a social X-ray like none other for how the country really felt about women's physical strength. And how it felt was extremely ambivalent.

In 1980, *Sports Illustrated*'s Dan Levin wrote: "It's a ghastly portent to some: bodybuilding for women, one more step on the road to androgyny. It raises complex questions, and it strikes at deeply held values. Should women be bodybuilders at all, and if so, should they strive to look like firm Miss Americas or female versions of Arnold Schwarzenegger? And, of course, there is the concept of femininity—are large muscles feminine, does that matter, and what does 'femininity' mean, anyway?"

Many Americans—men and women—had a visceral reaction to women with *any* visible muscle, even women as otherwise conventionally feminine as Lisa Lyon. "There are still millions of women . . . trying to pour themselves into Calvin Klein jeans who would take one look at Lisa Lyon's lats and yelp in horror," noted *The Washington Post* in 1980.

When Lisa's mother learned her daughter was training with

Arnold Schwarzenegger, she half joked that Lisa should "change her name to avoid embarrassing the family."

For all of these reasons, before the seventies, Americans were rarely exposed to women who flaunted their muscle. In their seminal book on women's bodybuilding, *Pumping Iron II: The Unprecedented Woman*, Charles Gaines and George Butler point out that for most of human history, depictions of ripped women were almost nonexistent. "Though standards of beauty for women have historically varied more often and more radically than those for men," they write, "it is difficult to find muscular women celebrated or even recorded anywhere in written or visual history." After seeing his first truly cut woman on stage, the renowned bodybuilder Frank Zane, awestruck, remarked to a bystander: "You familiar with Carl Jung? Well, I don't think there's an archetype for this."

In the early twentieth century, if you *did* want to spot a strong woman, your best bet was to attend the circus, which featured performers with seemingly superhuman brawn. These women, pale and stern and physically imposing in their Victorian leotards, had monikers like Minerva, Vulcana, and Athleta. The most famous was the Austrian-born Katie Sandwina—a stage name she adopted after she outlifted the most famous strong *man* at the time, Eugen Sandow. Sandwina was a headliner with Ringling Bros. and Barnum & Bailey's Greatest Show on Earth who broke chains, juggled cannonballs, and lifted three men at a time to cheering crowds.*

The thirties saw the rise of Southern California's Muscle Beach, a stretch of sand in Santa Monica where tanned and smiling bodybuilders,

---

* Incidentally, the circus fostered a strikingly feminist culture. Many of its women performers had shunned conventional lives and become financially independent, emboldening them to speak up about women's equality. "In 1912, Sandwina became vice president of Barnum & Bailey's eight-hundred-member suffrage group," writes Haley Shapley in *Strong Like Her*, helping to earn women the right to vote.

gymnasts, and acrobats would demonstrate feats of strength and defy gravity as crowds gawked.

Muscle Beach gave rise to some of the biggest names in mid-century fitness, from Jack LaLanne to Joe Gold, the founder of Gold's Gym, where Lisa Lyon would pump iron decades later. But one of its brightest stars was a woman—a dazzling blonde named Abbye "Pudgy" Stockton who would prove to be many years ahead of her time.

Pudgy—a cheeky childhood nickname, since she was diminutive—was initially turned on to weightlifting by her boyfriend-turned-husband, Les Stockton, an upbeat UCLA grad and fixture on Muscle Beach. After high school, Pudgy took a job working as a telephone switchboard operator. Sitting all day, she began to gain weight. She told Les she wanted to slim down, and he suggested she try exercising with a set of barbells.

Like Lisa, Pudgy loved the way training with weights made her feel—and she began to get strong. Soon she joined Les on the beach, where they would put on exhibitions. In one act, she stood on the palm of Les's raised hand while pressing a 100-pound barbell overhead. Then they switched places, and she held *him* above *her* head.

Sparkly and shapely with a palpable sexuality, Pudgy appeared on dozens of magazine covers throughout the thirties and forties, offering a new model for what a beautiful woman could look like. She eventually opened one of the first-ever women's gyms, a small studio on Sunset Boulevard called the Salon of Figure Development; later, she and Les opened his and her gyms in Beverly Hills. For nearly a decade, she wrote a column for *Strength & Health* magazine called Barbelles, through which she aimed to inspire regular women to lift. Pudgy's business card read: *Foremost Female Physical Culturist—Writer, Authority on Feminine Figure Contouring, Cover Girl.*

But it would be decades before American women would start to lift en masse, or even to consider weights an acceptable tool for "figure contouring." Back then, *Sports Illustrated*'s Levin writes, "women's bodybuilding, 1980 style, was unimaginable."

The shift began with the rise of the women's movement, whose leaders understood that for women to feel truly equal to men, they had to feel physically equal. As early as 1971, *Our Bodies, Ourselves* suggested women "use dumbbells to build up arm, shoulder and torso muscles." (Women can work out with light hand weights, the authors note, but bench-pressing heavy metal is "more exciting.") The movement also encouraged women to train in self-defense—without the ability to protect their bodies, how could they enjoy the rights for which they were fighting? Women across the country began signing up for martial arts and other courses in physical combat.

In 1972, there was the watershed passage of Title IX. The law gave hundreds of thousands of young women access to serious athletic training facilities for the first time—including weight rooms. Many of these student athletes, observing how their male counterparts trained, started lifting to complement their own conditioning. After graduation, some continued to seek out facilities to lift, to keep challenging themselves to hold on to the strength they had built. But not all considered themselves feminists; they simply liked feeling strong.

By the end of the decade, women were lifting in greater numbers than ever before. Newspaper stories about women who had taken up lifting abounded. "Weightlifting gives you confidence in yourself," a twenty-something furniture saleswoman told *The Washington Post*. "You don't have to run and get a man every time there's a tough jar to open (or a sofa to move)." A young mother told the *Minneapolis Star*: "Men have been doing this for a long time, and there's no reason why women can't develop their muscles, too. Whether it's outwardly or inwardly, it's nice to like yourself both ways. That's what it's done for me. I feel proud when I look at the mirror." Plus, she said, when you're strong, "everything is easier."

Some of these women felt so proud of their new physiques they entered the country's first bodybuilding competitions. Others became unapologetic powerlifters. But many still feared that muscle would strip them of their femininity. That's where Lisa Lyon stepped in.

————————————

Lisa insisted in interviews that she wasn't a "women's libber," but she nonetheless championed a more expansive view of femininity—one in which female power was beautiful. The media ate it up. Publications from *Vogue* and *Rolling Stone* to *Esquire* profiled Lisa. David Letterman and Merv Griffin invited her onto their shows. NBC signed her as an on-camera bodybuilding commentator, and she began hawking a line of perfume, LISA, sold in a glass bottle shaped like a fist. With every appearance, she would make the case that visible muscle was not inherently masculine.

"The 1980s is the era of total womanhood—single girl, working wife and mother or whatever," she told a reporter. "Part of fulfilling that mission is a really healthy, well-developed body which will allow women to move freely in society and take whatever jobs she wants." She told another: "As far as long-term goals, I would like to show women that they can do things they 'aren't supposed to do.'" She bought tubes of liquid graphite, normally used to lubricate locks, from a hardware store to highlight the contours of her muscles on camera.

In 1981, the same year Jane Fonda published her original Workout book, Lisa wrote an exercise guide called *Lisa Lyon's Body Magic* to inspire regular women to train with weights. On the cover, she poses in a tank top and short shorts, holding a barbell behind her head. Open the book, and there is Lisa balancing Arnold Schwarzenegger, the epitome of manliness, on her trim shoulders.

She grew to relish being a provocateur, and in 1980, she posed nude for *Playboy*. "The fact is, I didn't need another picture in *Muscle Magazine*," she said of her decision. "The people who read *Playboy* are the ones that need to be educated to this concept of femininity." (Gloria Steinem later noted, "whether this was a victory for female muscle or for that magazine's traditional effort to show all women as sexually available was unclear.")

After *Playboy*, she posed nude for the high-fashion photographer Helmut Newton. And in 1983, the photographer Robert Mapplethorpe, whose previous muses had included iconoclasts such as Patti Smith and Debbie Harry, published an entire book of mostly erotic photos of Lisa. Coyly titled *Lady*, it featured dozens of black-and-white portraits that played on common (and some less common) tropes. There was Lisa as "bride, broad, doll, moll, playgirl, beach-girl, bike-girl, gym-girl, and boy-girl"; "as frog-person, mud-person, flamenco dancer, spiritist medium, archetypical huntress, circus artiste, snake-woman, society woman, young Christian, and kink." In essence: She was Everywoman.

Lisa's posing and proselytizing was working. Mainstream pop culture had begun to embrace the concept of women's weight training, and more women were pursuing both strength and Lisa's "contoured" figure. A growing roster of beautiful women bodybuilders were entering the spotlight, too, amplifying her message. A born-again Christian from Texas named Rachel McLish with soap-opera good looks soon rivaled Lisa in fame, as she parlayed her victories into book deals, product endorsements, posters, TV commercials—and eventually, a workout wear line at Kmart.

Some women were surely inspired by the 1983 movie *Flashdance*, in which actress Jennifer Beals lifts weights at a gym while chasing her dream of becoming a professional ballerina. Or by the women's magazines, from *Vogue* to *Cosmopolitan*, that featured bodybuilders' secrets for becoming strong and shapely. Or by the emerging scientific studies suggesting weight-bearing exercise promoted skeletal health in women. For women who felt intimidated by freestanding barbells, strength-training machines such as the Nautilus offered another route to muscle.

In 1981, the sibling publishers of *Muscle & Fitness*—Canadian brothers Joe and Ben Weider, two founders of modern men's bodybuilding—launched *Shape*, the first magazine devoted to women's strength and fitness. The magazine was conceived of by Joe Weider's wife, a bodybuilder and model named Betty Weider. The first issue featured the reigning Miss America on its cover, sheathed in a purple catsuit. Every issue after that boasted a celebrity cover model—a move Betty hoped would both continue to popularize exercise and satisfy women's increasingly insatiable desire to know the intimate details of professionally beautiful women's fitness regimens.

Publications geared toward Black women began to promote weightlifting, too, especially when, by the early eighties, bodybuilding began to produce Black champions. Most famous among them was a former competitive synchronized swimmer from New Jersey named Carla Dunlap, who in 1983 became the first Black woman to win the Ms. Olympia title—bodybuilding's highest honor. *Essence* celebrated Carla throughout the mid-eighties and shared her fitness advice with readers. "Body building makes you feel strong, so you're physically capable of doing a lot . . . and that changes your attitude about yourself," she told that magazine's readers in a 1985 feature titled "Getting Strong: Your Guide to Mental, Emotional, and Physical Power."

When we spoke for this book, Carla told me, "I always liked that I could ask my body to do anything and it would respond. I wouldn't have to sit there and go, 'Can I do this?' I would be like, 'Okay, let's try this. If I can't do it, maybe I can master it.'" When *Essence* featured her, readers wrote letters to the editor hailing her as their hero.

A decade earlier, a young Black strength coach named Henry McGhee had helped to create modern women's bodybuilding as a sport, full stop. In the early seventies, McGhee advocated for women's strength training through his post as associate physical director of the YMCA in Canton, Ohio, located in a predominantly Black neighborhood. He was inspired by his older sister, Tammy, a fantastic athlete who had been discouraged from participating in sports because she was a girl. "It just seemed wrong to me," he later said.

McGhee began training a few women in a special weight room at the Y created just for them, and in 1978, he organized what is believed to be the first bodybuilding competition in which women were judged on their muscularity, calling it the National Women's Physique Championships. "Women are incredible," he told *Sports Illustrated.* "We've just never seen them reach their potential."

By the summer of 1982, *Time* magazine ran a cover story titled "Coming on Strong" that declared muscle "the new beauty ideal." Inside, the film critic Richard Corliss writes: "You've come a long way, sister. . . . In the old days, when women's shapes were expected to be either pillows or posts, today's muscular woman might have been considered a freak. No more."

And yet. While America's acceptance of a more muscular, visibly strong female physique was a step forward, not all women's muscle was created equal. The muscular figures that pop culture idolized in the first half of the eighties looked a lot like Lisa Lyon—or Jane Fonda. They were bodies devoid of any apparent fat and the softness that had long defined womanhood. They were bodies that were still, by most metrics, small. And they were bodies that were mostly white.

While Carla Dunlap was an idol among Black women, celebrated for her beauty and brains as much as her strength, Joe and Ben Weider, the bodybuilding power brokers who ran an empire of fitness publications, refused to feature her on the covers of their magazines, and she was denied the TV commercials in which her white peers had begun to star. "I would win a contest and they would put the third-place person on the cover," Carla told me. "It was sort of this, 'Well, you know, you don't sell magazines,' or 'You're not pretty enough.'"

Meanwhile, the same mainstream women's magazines that sold tips for building muscle still featured only super thin models in the rest of their pages, sending a decidedly mixed message.

Even Lisa Lyon, for all her progressive views, stopped short of advocating for "massive" muscle. She spoke disparagingly about women who got "too big," telling *The Washington Post*, "you're not condemned to develop some gross, caricatured body just because you work out with weights," adding, "I don't want to criticize them if that's their idea of beauty; beauty is a subjective evaluation. But I don't want that. So it's a matter of stopping."

This perspective eventually led her to stop her activism, too. "I started this sport," she claimed, bluntly and hyperbolically, in 1981. "It's not my fault other women want to take it further."

The first few years of the eighties indeed saw, as *Sports Illustrated*'s Dan Levin put it, the birth of a niche class of what some would call "female Arnold Schwarzeneggers"—women bodybuilders who strove to get as big, and as strong, as possible. In a 1983 essay in *Vogue* titled "Tough Women," writer Kay Larson tells of a secret desire she and her friends shared to be "so gleefully, gratifyingly musclebound." But few women would ever act on such a desire. Because while *some* female muscle was attractive, "too much" was still *too much*.

The game had changed, but the rules were the same: Less was still more for women.

When NBC agreed to broadcast women's bodybuilding in the early eighties, executives told contest organizers that while they'd love for the really massive women to get a lot of time onstage—TV viewers were fascinated by them—under no circumstances could one of them win.

The era saw another major fitness innovation that would both support and complicate women's pursuit of muscle: Gyms became co-ed. *Cue up the disco music.*

For decades, men and women had exercised in separate facilities or on alternate days. Polite society considered sweating in mixed company improper—besides, so few adult women *wanted* to sweat at gyms that many gyms didn't even have a women's restroom or locker room. The few women's gyms that did exist still offered vibrating belts and rolling machines. But with the rise of running and aerobics and strength-training, more women sought out memberships. And this demand helped to fuel the rise of the co-ed, multipurpose gyms and health clubs—sprawling facilities where you could run on a treadmill, cycle on an exercise bike, take aerobics class, swim laps, play a game of racquetball, use a Nautilus machine or lift weights, and grab some carrot juice at the juice bar on your way out. And, of course, schmooze with fellow gym-goers.

Fitness historians note that, in the seventies and early eighties, gyms became what the sociologist Ray Oldenburg termed a "third place"—a place outside of home and office to meet and hang out with like-minded people, a place central to community life, and often, to one's identity. For centuries, houses of worship had served this purpose. But with organized religion on the decline, gyms began to take their place, "with sweating their form of prayer," noted journalist Blair Sabol in her 1986 book *The Body of America: An Insider's Journey Through the Bumps & Pumps, Groans & Moans, Pecs &*

Wrecks, Sweat & Sex of the Fitness Explosion. "At least in these places of worship cursing is allowed," she jokes. "But please, no smoking."

Gyms soon took on a reputation as the country's new singles bars. "Health clubs aren't just clubs; they have become communities that present a fantasy of beauty and fitness that's within reach," Sabol writes. "Which is why in the early 1980s, they also became a fantasy pickup palace." *Rolling Stone* writer Aaron Latham immortalized gyms' new role in a feature for the magazine titled "Looking for Mr. Goodbody," a play on the title of Judith Rossner's bestselling 1975 novel and the 1977 film *Looking for Mr. Goodbar.* The series focused specifically on a swinging L.A. health club called the Sports Connection.

"At the bars, you look like you're just waiting to meet somebody," one member told Latham. "At a health club, at least you have an excuse to be there. You don't look so obvious."

Another woman chimed in: "It's an alternative to the disco era. Now it's not fashionable to go to a disco, but it is fashionable to go to a health club. It's a socially acceptable way of meeting someone. You could tell your mother."

What did this mean for women's pursuit of strength? It meant that at the same time women gained easy access to barbells, dumbbells, bench presses, and weight machines, going to the gym became entangled with attracting and looking for a man. In the most jaundiced view, it meant women were suddenly in direct sexual competition with one another on the gym floor.

Naturally, adapting to the cultural moment they found themselves in, women began getting decked out to work out. Leotards, once a garment of liberation, became increasingly sexy. They began featuring what Sabol dubbed the "high-intensity crotch"—a groin area with legs cut so high, I shudder thinking about what must have happened when one of its wearers hopped on a stationary bike. "To be even a passable model for such a garment," writes Sabol, "you either had to be eight years old or have an all-over body wax."*

A 1983 *New York Times* feature chronicled this rising trend of "sweat chic." At a health club in midtown Manhattan, the paper reported, a thirty-two-year-old graphic designer worked out "wearing a satiny red leotard cut high on the thighs and low in the back, a white headband, shimmery white tights, black wool leg warmers, a thin black belt around her waist and a gold Egyptian necklace." The woman explains: "I work out every day of the week . . . and when I look good, I work harder."

For women who wanted to exercise without being ogled, the era also saw the rise of the multipurpose women's gym. In 1969, a savvy Eastern European immigrant named Lucille Roberts opened one of the first and most successful of these gyms, originally housed in a small space across from New York City's iconic Macy's department store.

Roberts's family was Jewish, and she was born in the Soviet Union in what is now an independent country, Tajikistan. Facing religious persecution in the Soviet Union, her family immigrated to the United States and settled in Flatbush, Brooklyn, when she was thirteen. After graduating from college in 1964 and working in retail for a few years, she decided she wanted to work for herself. She was an early adopter of exercise—a "self-described exercise nut"—and she "hated to deal with inventory," according to *The New York Times*. So she and her husband invested their savings in what became the first Lucille Roberts women's gym.

Roberts's target clientele was women who didn't have the time or money to visit one of the city's exclusive women's health spas or

---

* *Gymnasium* does come from the Greek word *gymnos*, which means "nude," after all. In antiquity, Greek men would strip down and cover themselves in oil before working out. Which, frankly, sounds more comfortable than exercising with a "high-intensity crotch."

studios: secretaries, teachers, the wives of policemen, and other middle-class women "with two kids and two jobs" who wanted to work up a quick sweat on their way to Penn Station and be on the train by six o'clock. "It was like coming out with hamburgers when nobody else was making hamburgers," Roberts once said. The original gym soon grew into a mini-empire throughout the region.

Roberts's timing was impeccable: The gyms would thrive in the seventies, bolstered by the push for women's empowerment. Given the era, wrote the *Times*'s Susan Dominus, "a gathering of women inevitably had the whiff of empowerment, and Roberts noticed." The gyms started offering classes in self-defense, classes in how to report an abusive husband, classes in how to install a burglar alarm. Later, Roberts chose to keep the gyms women-only because "I don't want to get undressed, put on a thong and work out in front of a bunch of men."

But Roberts's feminist enlightenment had its limits. In 1997, she told *The New York Times*: "It is only the upper classes who are into exercise for health. . . . The middle classes just want to look good. We have tried health classes. They just want to fit into tight jeans."

Feminist or not, Roberts's approach was so successful that she, her husband, and their two kids eventually moved into the former Woolworth mansion off Fifth Avenue.

The gym model that would take over America, however, was the one that sizzled with sexual tension. And this model, like the larger fitness industry, was predominantly white.

Since the modern fitness movement's earliest days, many clubs—including YMCAs in white neighborhoods—discriminated against nonwhite prospective members, writes historian Shelly McKenzie in *Getting Physical*. Throughout the mid-twentieth century, "[taking] their cues from country clubs, both commercial and nonprofit clubs worked to ensure that their membership was composed of 'desirable clients,'" writes McKenzie, engaging in racial and religious profiling.

Gyms continued to discriminate based on race through the eighties. In one particularly egregious example, McKenzie continues, the Justice Department in 1989 filed a civil suit against the owner of a health club chain called Holiday Spa that operated health clubs in Washington, Baltimore, Philadelphia, Boston, and Atlanta. The suit alleged that employees were told to "discourage black customers from joining and quoted them higher rates and poorer credit terms than those offered to white customers." Groups of club members and employees brought additional suits against U.S. Health, charging that prospective Black members were coded in internal documents as "DNWAM," or "do not want as member." In 1991 the chain admitted guilt, and as part of a settlement, paid damages and offered free memberships to Black customers who had paid inflated rates or had been denied access to the clubs.

This level of blatant discrimination, combined with the "cultural profile of the typical exerciser as a white professional," helps to explain the relative absence of Black Americans from the decade's fitness trends. As *Sports Illustrated* noted in 1984: "You can scan hundreds of product catalogs, mail-order brochures, fitness magazines, books and videos and see nothing but attractive lily-white faces."

There were subtler forms of racism in fitness, too.

In 1982, the beloved Jane Fonda Workout instructor Janice Darling struck out on her own to open an aerobics studio in Culver City called the Sweat Shop, where she continued to encourage students to cultivate mental as well as physical strength through rigorous workouts.

For a few years, the studio was a phenomenon, earning press in local and national publications. And yet, Janice remembers, writers often described her studio using racially loaded language. "They would say it was 'tribal' or it was 'raw,'" she told me. "They gave it a Black connotation—it kind of had a jungle aspect to it."

Janice hoped to parlay her popularity among L.A. locals into a fitness video, which could offer her a much-needed source of additional income. But the opportunities never came. "As a Black woman, I never got the fame or publicity of a Kathy Smith or a Richard Simmons," she told me. "[People] used to call me the Tina Turner of fitness. But they didn't want the Tina Turner of fitness. They wanted the Kathy Smith of fitness."

———————

It was only a matter of time before Hollywood found inspiration in the gym scene, capitalizing on its outsize sexed-up role in white middle-class Americans' life. In 1984, Aaron Latham's *Rolling Stone* series was adapted into a feature film called *Perfect*, starring John Travolta and Jamie Lee Curtis. (The film, which was a colossal flop, includes an astonishing five-minute-long aerobics sequence in which Curtis, playing an instructor, locks eyes with Travolta, while they bump and thrust their pelvises to the beat in a simulated sex scene.) There was *Getting Physical*, a made-for-TV movie about a woman who loses weight and gains self-esteem by lifting weights, which features Lisa Lyon in a bit part. And ABC aired the short-lived *Shaping Up*, a sitcom about a gang of gym employees, starring Leslie Nielsen, Michael Fontaine, and Jennifer Tilly.

But the pop culture offering that became emblematic not only of the fitness explosion but also the decade itself was Olivia Newton-John's smash hit "Physical."

The story behind "Physical" is largely one of happenstance. Initially, the song wasn't intended to be about working out at all. It was only about sex.

The British-Australian songwriting duo Terry Shaddick and Steve Kipner had written the song for Tina Turner, but when the Queen of Rock heard the racy lyrics, she decided it was too sexual for her—what with lines about "bringing out the animal in her" and all. Turner and Newton-John shared a manager, and Turner suggested he offer it instead to the Australian singer, who was best known at the time for her role as the wholesome Sandy in 1978's *Grease.*

Olivia Newton-John instantly loved the song. She was bored with ballads, and it was so catchy! So she flew to L.A. to record it. Then she panicked.

"Maybe it was too raunchy?" she remembers thinking.

"The lyrics had me singing: 'There's nothing left to talk about unless it's horizontally!'" she wrote in her memoir, *Olivia Newton-John: Don't Stop Believin'.* What would people think?

These were the very early days of MTV and music videos, and Newton-John's manager had persuaded her to create a video for every song on her upcoming album. She had an idea: Why not suggest the song was about exercise? "Maybe if we redefined the idea of getting physical, it would take on a whole new meaning," she told him. "We can take the focus off the other part . . . Sort of like a double entendre."

The rest is pop history. The music video for "Physical" stars Newton-John as the sole female exerciser in a gym full of half-naked, out-of-condition men whom she attempts to whip into shape. (The blatant fat-shaming baked into this story line was standard fare in the eighties.) Her look—torn teal-blue T-shirt over a white leotard and hot pink tights, paired with a white headband—would help to inspire the workout-themed look of the decade.

At the end of the video, the men, who have been working up a sweat on stationary bikes and rowing machines and weight machines, emerge as calendar-worthy studs. Then, in a surprise twist, two of the guys fall for each other and walk out of the gym hand in hand. (This was both progressive and a relic of the not-so-long-ago past, when Americans raised a homophobic eyebrow at any man who devoted "too much" time to shaping his physique.)

When the "Physical" video debuted on ABC on February 8, 1982, more than a third of America's TV-watching audience tuned in. (Notably, ABC cut the video's gay finale for its broadcast.) The single rocketed to number one on *Billboard*'s pop chart. And the video won a Grammy for Video of the Year.

Later, *Billboard* declared "Physical" the number one pop hit of the eighties.

Fitness had always relied on the promise of aesthetic transformation as an incentive. But in the eighties, a fit body became more than just a beautiful body. The fit body became a symbol—of discipline, determination, and drive. "To be in condition is not only healthy, it is sexy—and inseparable from a strength of the self and the spirit," *Time*'s Richard Corliss declared.

It was during this era that a fit body became a defining goal of American life, a *way* of life, the ultimate capitalist status symbol. It girded the great Reagan-era myth, writes Susan J. Douglas, "that superficial appearances really can be equated with a person's deepest character strengths and weaknesses." The myth would stick, driving Americans to pour billions of dollars into the fitness and wellness industries to this day.

Middle- and upper-class Americans' wardrobes became increasingly dominated by activewear, as signaling that one cared about working out was as important as actually working out (another trend that lives on). "Now all the world was a gym and our closets were fast becoming lockers," wrote Blair Sabol. "In fact, jock couture was probably the first time American designers became an honest fashion force. We had *the handle* on sweat and lifestyle, while Europe continued to runway sleek and fantasy."

Throughout the eighties, as more women got strong, the ante for acceptable levels of women's muscle also continued to be upped. In 1987, Jane Fonda produced her first workout video using free weights. The same year, Kathy Smith published *Winning Workout*, a book devoted to exercising with free weights. The end of the decade saw the emergence of celebrity trainers—personal trainers to the rich and famous who then became rich and famous themselves. Madonna, the era's uber-influencer, proudly showed off an increasingly buff physique.

But arguably the biggest leap forward for women's muscle during this time again happened alongside Arnold Schwarzenegger. (He'll be back?) In her reprisal of the role of Sarah Connor in 1991's *Terminator 2: Judgment Day*, Linda Hamilton caused jaws to drop when she bared her guns on screen. Her arms weren't just toned; they were *powerful*. Deeply defined and sinewy with muscle—a radical departure not only from her physique in the original film but from the bodies of virtually every actress in Hollywood at the time.

Even Arnold was impressed. "Linda, you are ripped to shreds," he reportedly told her.

By then, women's muscle had been sufficiently normalized that instead of balking at her arms, women wanted them. Personal trainers were flooded with requests from clients to help sculpt their biceps in her image. America still considered "too much" muscle freakish, but the bar was gradually rising. Among women, powerful arms became, as one *New York Times* contributor put it, like "a signal to one another that they are superwomen." (Nearly two decades later, First Lady Michelle Obama would inspire a similar arm lust.)

And so it came to be, as these social and cultural shifts converged, that American Everywomen from teens through the middle-aged grew to desire bodies of steel—and Tamilee Webb, a one-time body-builder and Everywoman herself, became a home video superstar.

————————

Tamilee Webb grew up on a farm in the small Northern California town of Rio Dell—or "Real Dull," as she and her friends joked. With an older half brother, two younger brothers, and mostly male cousins, she spent her childhood running around outside, playing sports and games, and proving she could keep up with the boys. ("I didn't own one doll," she told me in an interview. "No one wanted to play dolls!") If the boys wanted to get under her skin, all they had to do was tease her about her most notable feature: *Bubble Butt!* they'd yell.

When she got tired of her brothers, Tamilee adored spending time with her dad, who had been a star baseball player in their community as a young man. He encouraged her to pursue an education along with her dream of becoming a country singer and told her she could be whatever she wanted to be in life.

When she was fourteen, tragedy struck: Her dad, only thirty-seven years old, died of an undiagnosed heart defect while coaching one of her brothers' Little League games.

Over the next several years, Tamilee felt lost, overcome by grief. But she found solace in her physical strength. Eventually, after a few years of junior college, she enrolled at California State University at Chico, where she majored in physical education and later completed a graduate degree in exercise science.

It was at Chico, around 1980, that she first ventured into a weight room—becoming the first woman *welcomed* into the school's weight room. Initially, she told me, "the guys were not very receptive to it. But when they realized I was serious, and I asked them for help and various things, they all became like my big brothers."

Tamilee was inspired by Lisa Lyon and other early bodybuilding stars who projected beauty and femininity, and she decided to enter women's bodybuilding contests as part of her graduate research. "I wanted to see if bodybuilding biochemically damaged a woman's body," she said—or, really, to help disprove the still-pervasive belief that weightlifting would "turn a woman into a man." She was happy to be a guinea pig.

In the weight room, Tamilee developed her biceps and abdominals. She also focused on the region of her body that had always made her self-conscious: her thighs and butt.

She loved knowing she was becoming stronger and stronger. At an early bodybuilding contest, she didn't win any major prizes, but she did score an award for "best poser." And she was happy to report to her graduate advisers that she had suffered no ill effects.

Tamilee entered a few more competitions, but she didn't see a future for herself as a professional bodybuilder. But what *were* her options, with degrees in exercise? She could become a phys ed teacher—for decades, PE teacher was one of the few career opportunities that existed for women who wanted to turn an interest in fitness into a profession. But the notion didn't light a fire in her. She had heard about the burgeoning fitness scene in Southern California, and while she wasn't especially drawn to aerobic dance, either, she became hopeful she could find work in the land of bikinis, beaches, and bodies beautiful. "I wanted to help people stay fit and healthy and show them, look, you can lift weights and you're not going to look like a guy."

At twenty-three, Tamilee drove down to San Diego with her cocker spaniel/poodle mix, Tigger, in the passenger seat of her Toyota Celica. Once she arrived—with few friends in the area and a pet in tow—she was forced to live in her car for a couple weeks until she could get on her feet. "You do what you gotta do when you're young," she told me.

She began applying for jobs at local exercise facilities until finally she caught her big break. The owner of the chichi Golden Door Health Spa—the same owner who had given Jazzercise's Judi Sheppard Missett her first job in San Diego—offered to hire her to be a private trainer for her upscale clientele, who shelled out thousands of dollars a week to stay at the spa.

Tamilee would get paid five dollars an hour.

The Golden Door proved to be just that for Tamilee—a gateway, introducing her to a steady stream of VIPs. Her very first client was the model Christie Brinkley—an auspicious start, she thought. (Brinkley would eventually release her own fitness book and videos.)

Another client was married to a literary agent, who would help propel her to national fame.

Tamilee had begun incorporating a large rubber band into her workouts—she had snagged it from a physical therapist's office—and her client loved exercising with it. Not only did it build strength, you could pack it in a suitcase and take it anywhere!

One thing led to another, and thanks to her enthusiastic client, Tamilee landed a book deal with Workman Publishing. In 1986, she published the *Rubber Band Workout*, with a foreword by the *Today* show's on-air "family doctor," Dr. Art Ulene.

Workman sent Tamilee on a massive cross-country publicity tour, through which she caught the eye of more decision makers in the fitness industry—including those at a small video production and distribution company looking for a woman to front a new video series. The company had one very important requirement: The woman must have a "good butt."

The *Buns of Steel* brand initially began in Alaska. The original video starred an aerobics studio owner and former competitive pole vaulter named Greg Smithey. The story goes like this: One day after class in his Anchorage studio, a student told Smithey—who bore a striking resemblance to the actor Chuck Norris, complete with the headband—that his buns were fantastic.

In fact, she said, he had—*dun dun dun*—buns of steel.

Greg Smithey knew marketing gold when he heard it. He set to work producing a low-budget video that he called *Buns of Steel*. The video features Smithey leading a class of students (almost all women) through a routine of lower body strengthening and toning exercises that grew out of his pole-vaulting training.

A small New York–based distribution company called the Maier Group acquired the rights to the video, and not long after its release in 1987, it began to move copies. The tape saw particularly robust sales in San Francisco, where it became a hot commodity among the city's gay population.

Eventually, Maier Group executives wanted to build on the brand, and they wanted a woman to front it.

They found their star in Tamilee.

Tamilee offered a kind of bridge between women bodybuilders and everyday weight trainers. She was more muscular than many other female fitness personalities at the time, but her muscles were petite and compact. She was conventionally feminine and approachable-looking, appearing on camera in a sports bra, bikini bottoms, and nude tights (leotards were on the way out), her blond hair teased and scrunchied into a high half-ponytail. She also possessed the required buns of steel.

The video was no six-figure Jane Fonda production. Shot in Denver, Colorado, on a shoestring budget, it featured Tamilee in front of a glass-brick wall as she walked viewers through a rigorous series of butt and thigh-strengthening exercises. No frills, just squats.

Tamilee agreed to be paid pennies, but she insisted that her body and name appear on the front and back of the box. "I'm thinking, all right, I'm trying to build my career and want to do more of these," she told me. "I didn't want to be just talent."

It was a good choice on everyone's part. With Tamilee's glistening body now on the box, free weights in hand, sales were even more robust.

"I did one, and it just took off," she told me. Soon after that first tape, released in 1991, the Maier Group tapped Tamilee to make *Abs of Steel* and *Arms of Steel*. "And then they came back and said, 'We want you to do three more.'" By 1993, Tamilee's videos claimed six out of twenty slots on *Billboard*'s Health and Fitness home video chart.

The first time Tamilee appeared on the home-shopping network QVC to promote the *Steel* series, the network sold out of its inventory in five minutes. The tapes lined shelves at Blockbuster video stores and Kmarts and other retailers nationwide, with the tagline "Now you can have the buns you've always wanted."

By the late nineties, Tamilee's *Steel* videos had sold more than 10 million copies, and Tamilee herself had become a fixture in living rooms from coast to coast, starring in a total of twenty-two of the franchise's videos. And she'd earned a small fortune along the way.

As much as American women had been conditioned to long for what Tamilee was selling, many also recognized its absurdism. Throughout the decade, the dream of having body parts of steel became fodder for comic strips and butts of jokes. In the 1995 teen comedy *Clueless*, Cher (Alicia Silverstone) earnestly recommends Tamilee's workout in her attempt to teach her new friend and mentee, Tai (Brittany Murphy), how to be a desirable woman. After three minutes of squats, Tai laments, "My buns, they don't feel nothin' like steel!"

Later in the decade, a volume of *Cathy* cartoons paid homage to the series, with the title *Abs of Steel, Buns of Cinnamon*—in which Cathy puzzles over how to achieve this new standard for women. *ACK!*, to quote Cathy's favorite catchphrase.

But the promise was too powerful for many women to resist.

Striving for bodies of steel undoubtedly provided women with a new level of everyday strength. Stronger abdominal, arm, leg, and glute muscles allow a woman to navigate daily life with greater ease—and as she ages, with fewer aches and pains. They enhance her quality of life.

But for every cultural action, there is a reaction—and the rise of women's muscle brought a whammy of a backlash. With the explosion of the larger fitness movement and the notion that a fit body was a virtuous body, striving for a body of steel began to be presented not so much like a *choice* and more like a requirement of womanhood; a steel trap, if you will. Because along with striving for visible muscles, women were also simultaneously encouraged to strive for as little body fat as possible. Pop culture sent the message that having a body of steel didn't mean looking like a competitive bodybuilder so much as looking impossibly hard and lean.

While women's fitness culture at its best could offer women control over their bodies, it increasingly *demanded* that women control their bodies—to achieve one highly specific physical ideal.

Throughout the eighties, with more women pursuing careers than ever before, the feminine mystique of the fifties and sixties that glorified housework was replaced by a glorification of beauty work, as popular media and advertisers redoubled their efforts to capitalize on women's physical insecurities. Women were encouraged to address their "problem areas"—parts of the body that stubbornly held on to fat deposits. Workout videos became increasingly focused on "spot toning"—strategically working each major muscle group one at a time, with the presumed goal of eventually perfecting them all—dooming women to a cycle of constantly striving for more (or less, as it were). These videos were also increasingly fronted by ultra-thin fashion models. It was only in the seventies that the cosmetics industry introduced the word *cellulite* into the cultural vocabulary as something women needed to fear and loathe; something that should make her feel worthless. A 1993 survey found that while only 6 percent of women wished their breasts were either bigger or smaller, nearly two-thirds wished they had "better thighs."

Even Lucille Roberts's gyms played a part in this cultural messaging: In 1989, the chain aired a TV commercial that showed a crowd fleeing from a movie theater as a blob "oozes menacingly through the doors," reported *The New York Times*. "In the background, a puckish narrator asks, 'Thighs getting out of control?'"

The same year Tamilee's *Buns of Steel* video was released, former *Three's Company* star Suzanne Somers released the ThighMaster—a resistance-based gadget that promised to help women "master" their otherwise uncontrollable bodies. In a doozy of an origin story, Somers had been inspired to enter the fitness business after she was unceremoniously let go from *Three's Company* because she demanded to be paid as much as her male costar. "The network decided to make an example of me so that no other woman would have the audacity to ask for parity," Somers told *Entrepreneur* magazine in 2020. "I lost that great job, and I was so devastated at the time, but life is about veiled gifts. I was suddenly kicked out on the streets, but I kept reinventing myself, and my husband and I decided we wouldn't work for anyone ever again." When approached with an early prototype of the ThighMaster, Somers and her husband saw an opportunity. They branded and began manufacturing the gizmo—and sold ten million units "right out the gate."

Indeed, throughout the eighties, the smooth, dimple-free thigh and butt became "the ultimate signifier of female fitness, beauty, and character," writes Susan J. Douglas in *Where the Girls Are*, published in 1994. "Perfect thighs, in other words, were an achievement, a product, and one to be admired and envied. They demonstrated that the woman had made something of herself, that she had character and class, that she was the master of her body and, thus, of her fate. If she had conquered her own adipose tissue, she could conquer anything. She was a new woman, liberated and in control."

It's no surprise that, throughout the eighties and nineties, eating disorder diagnoses soared. So did the number of women seeking plastic surgery. And eventually, the rise of women's muscle, lithe as it was, led the fashion industry to "reintroduce weakness," as Gloria Steinem put it, with its re-glorification of the hollow-eyed waif look. It was Twiggy all over again, in the form of supermodel Kate Moss—"but at least it's being protested," Steinem added.

─────────────

By the time I was a teenager in the mid-nineties, I didn't think much about exercising to become strong. I was a beneficiary of Title IX, and I ran a season of track and cross-country my freshman year of high school, but I was at the back of the pack. (Okay, behind the pack.) I didn't aspire to become athletic. I aspired to mold, refine, perfect my post-puberty body—which was decidedly less lean than my childhood body—into a conventionally beautiful one. Which meant a smaller one. And the now fully hatched fitness industrial complex offered me a cornucopia of resources promising to help me achieve this goal.

A child of the eighties, I had grown up playing with Mattel's Great Shape Barbie, who sported the not-so-subtle tagline: "She works out & looks great!" I coveted Hasbro's Get in Shape, Girl! workout sets—toy kits "for today's young girl" that included various combinations of exercise books, audiocassettes, and kid-sized workout equipment, including pastel hand weights, a ballet barre, and a floor mat. I remember how exercising to the tapes made me feel like a grown-up, in the same way wearing my mom's lipstick did. Working out, I gathered, was just what ladies *did*.

But I had the luxury of seeing Get in Shape, Girl! as simply a toy, because I was physically slim as a girl. When I mentioned Get in Shape, Girl! on social media while writing this book, an acquaintance sent me this note:

> I totally remember Get in Shape, Girl! and could sing the ad jingle for you. I grew up chubby and was overweight by college—precisely because I started dieting by fifth grade. I remember asking for it for my birthday or Christmas, thinking, This will be the thing that makes me "normal," by which I meant "thin." Of course it wasn't. It wasn't until I was in my late 20s and early 30s that I realized physical exercise didn't have to be punitive.

In middle school, my fitness bible was *Beauty and Fitness with Saved by the Bell*, a slim 1992 manual featuring inspiration from stars Tiffani-Amber Thiessen, Elizabeth Berkley, and Lark Voorhies. "Working out can be a total blast!" the book promises. "Elizabeth, Lark, and Tiffani all work out regularly, and they love it." I devoured issues of *Seventeen* and *YM* for tips on how to improve each region of my body, awkwardly attempting to follow along with the photo guides of sweatless, perfectly made-up teen girls exercising on neon-hued mats.

As I entered high school, I became most loyal to a workout series called The Firm (get it?). Night after night, I summoned a shirtless fitness model named Tracy James onto our old wood-paneled television and followed his advice, delivered in a thick Jersey accent, for developing six-pack abs. (Tracy James, I recently learned, was essentially just a well-developed hunk The Firm hired to host this particular video. He was later voted *Cosmopolitan*'s Man of the Year and also appeared on the covers of romance novels.) After absorbing his introduction to the concept of sit-ups, I followed along as nameless ladies in shiny leotards instructed me to reach, crunch, and tune into my abdominals, my ankles wrapped in weights.

I wanted muscle—badly. I wanted "well-defined" arms that, I thought, would look nice in tank tops. I wanted a firm "stomach." I wanted sleek thighs and a compact butt. (I spotted my first patches of cellulite around age sixteen.)

But muscle for strength? That was a fringe benefit. And I wasn't alone. What was once a bold feminist action had become, for many women, if not totally disconnected from the pursuit of strength, a secondary goal. It would be years before that would change for me— and for many American women.

———

In the last decade, however, things really *have* started to change, slowly but steadily. Women's bodybuilding remains a kind of side-show sport, tainted by rumors of steroids and a fundamental lack of understanding of *Why? Why would a woman feel compelled to get that big?* But there are signs of progress, evidenced perhaps most potently by the rise of CrossFit, the popular hard-core strength-building regimen whose devotees are nearly 50 percent women.

When women first show up to CrossFit, writes journalist J. C. Herz in *Learning to Breathe Fire: The Rise of CrossFit and the Primal Future of Fitness*, they balk at the prospect of someday becoming as large—as ripped—as the more seasoned female lifters. "But then two months go by, and these women decide they want to climb a rope or deadlift their bodyweight." And eventually, "their bodies become a by-product of what they're able to do."

Shannon Wagner, founder of the Women's Strength Coalition, a group dedicated to helping women and non-cisgender men cultivate muscle, described her experience with weight training this way: "For me, picking up a barbell meant focusing on my body, for the first time, in a way that had nothing to do with shrinking or making myself smaller. It felt radical to search for safety in myself, as opposed to looking for it in the approval from others. When I chose to stop getting smaller in my physical body, I stopped existing for other people."

Perhaps the 2020s will be the decade women finally make peace with taking up space. "For hundreds of years, women have been told that weakness is sexy," writes journalist Haley Shapley in her 2020 book *Strong Like Her*. "Men are supposed to be big and powerful. Women are dainty and beautiful. Blur those lines, and you might just be a man-hater, ugly, misguided, or all of the above. Until *bulky* is no longer the scariest descriptor that can be used in reference to a woman's body, we won't know what's truly possible."

Back in the nineties, meanwhile, many of the women who had started exercising in the seventies and eighties were starting to feel burnt out—from aerobics, from big-gym culture, from striving for bodies of steel, from existing for other people. Baby boomers had squarely hit middle age, and many suffered injuries from overdoing it or from following fitness leaders who didn't always know what they were doing. They had felt the burn and were ready to cool down.

And so, millions began to seek out a gentler approach to fitness. One that promised to restore their weary bodies—in some cases, their very souls.

CHAPTER 7

Stretch

Wanna fly, you got to give up the shit
that weighs you down.

—Toni Morrison

Yoga wasn't exactly new to the world when it exploded in America. Like an ever-present *om*, it had hummed in the background of the burgeoning fitness movement since its inception, unfurling like a lotus flower until the conditions were right for it to burst into full bloom. When it did, it would eventually propel millions of women to slip into Lululemons and bend, stretch, and breathe in the name of beauty, strength, and calm.

By the late eighties, waves of middle- and upper-class American women who had pushed their bodies to the max for years found that they were exhausted. They were working outside the home in record numbers while raising children—and trying to follow Jane Fonda's advice to never miss a day of exercise. *No excuses.* Many were nursing injuries borne from overuse. Some were disillusioned that exercise couldn't, as promised, completely override their genes and turn them *into* Jane Fonda. In *The Body of America*, journalist Blair Sabol counted herself among these weary women. "Basically, we all need a giant rest," she wrote. "We've pounded and pumped, humped, and dumped our physiques into a vacuum and now we need to get back to some sense of basics—to forms of moderate movement."

Despite the fact that women's body ideals now required more work than ever to achieve—or perhaps in *response* to this development— in the late eighties, the percentage of women who exercised was decreasing for the first time since the fifties. By the nineties, the trend had shaken the fitness industry. "After years of bowing to a hard-body ideal, fitness-conscious baby boomers are beginning to drop high-intensity gym regimens and embrace more leisurely activities," *AdAge* declared in 1994. Health club memberships were falling. Once-popular aerobics studios were shuttering. Even athletic shoe sales were flatlining.

Fewer men were exercising, too, but the decline was especially pronounced among women. "It's a response to the Superwomen phenomenon," the research director of the National Sporting Goods Association told *AdAge*, nodding to the burden society placed on women to do it all and have it all. "Something's got to give."

But what? Women had experienced the revelatory benefits of exercise, and most weren't ready to quit the habit entirely. *AdAge* noted that walking and gardening were growing in popularity and might even become the next fitness phenoms. Easy Spirit was seeing walking shoe sales rise—an exception to the broader shoe trend— and gardening glove sales were also picking up pace.

This was a nice thought, but most women still valued being part of a fitness community and appreciated having an excuse to leave the house. They still wanted an active way to shape their bodies. For many, the glamour and sex appeal of gym life had been motivating, and it's tough to imagine two less sexy activities than walking and gardening.

It was into this void that yoga would stretch—as an exercise regimen, beauty ritual, path to inner calm, lifestyle of the rich and famous, and multibillion-dollar industry. From 1990 to 2002, the number of Americans who practiced yoga at least three times a month grew from 4 million to more than 28 million. By 1994, both Jane Fonda and Kathy Smith had released yoga exercise videos. That same year a *U.S. News & World Report* cover declared that yoga had "gone mainstream." Celebrities from Madonna to Gwyneth Paltrow to Uma Thurman swore by it. And the vast majority of its devotees were women.

Like so many fitness movements before it, yoga might never have caught on among American women if it weren't for one intensely focused and doggedly determined woman.

To understand how yoga exploded in the nineties, we have to go back to where this book began—to an America whose middle- and upper-class white women were craving a sense of purpose and identity outside their roles as wives and mothers, despite the comforts of postwar life. While on the East Coast Bonnie Prudden was evangelizing about the benefits of breaking a sweat, a Russian actress named Indra Devi was setting up shop in Hollywood, where she would enthusiastically pitch yoga as an ancient antidote to America's "modern way of life."

Indra Devi, like so many fitness pioneers, was a master of self-reinvention. For starters, her name wasn't always Indra Devi. The daughter of a Swedish bank manager and a Russian noblewoman turned actress, she was born Eugenia Peterson in 1899 in Riga, Latvia, which was then part of the Russian empire. For a while she went by the anglicized name of Jane—and in many ways, she was a kind of cultural predecessor to the fitness world's *other* towering Jane. By the time she was in her forties, having long traded fur coats for saris, she would offer herself up as evidence that, through yoga, a woman could become whomever she wanted.

There's a reason why volumes have been written about Indra Devi, most notably Michelle Goldberg's 2015 biography, *The Goddess Pose: The Audacious Life of Indra Devi, the Woman Who Helped Bring Yoga to the West,* a deeply researched chronicle of her epic life. Before she arrived in Hollywood in 1947, Devi had already lived multiple "audacious" chapters. Like an "esoteric female Forrest Gump," writes Goldberg, she "seemed to show up wherever tumultuous world events were unfolding."

Physically small, Eugenia Peterson had an outsize sense of adventure. She wasn't conventionally beautiful, but there was something striking about her quietly determined face. She leveraged her looks and charisma to charm friends and lovers around the world—and later, to attract followers. "As a child, I intuited that happiness only came to those that dared to follow their own path," Devi wrote in her memoirs. "I forged myself as an independent being, and I was never tied to a place, nor a religion."

But Eugenia's life was fueled by more than just a spirit of independence. When she was a little girl, her young mother left her in the care of her grandparents for long stretches while she fled to pursue her own dreams of acting. Eugenia soon found herself struggling with anxiety. She was "plagued by inexplicable terrors," writes Goldberg. "She was afraid of death, afraid that her mother would die, terrified that her nanny would abandon her." She was especially afraid of being buried alive. The emotional challenges of her early life ignited a lifelong quest for spiritual comfort and guidance.

Eugenia first encountered the word *yoga* as a fifteen-year-old, while visiting one of her mother's actor friends in Moscow. There she wandered into the home's library and stumbled on a book titled *Fourteen Lessons in Yogi Philosophy and Oriental Occultism.* She picked it up, intrigued.

When the book's owner found Eugenia perched on a footstool and thumbing through the volume, he began reading passages aloud. She listened "breathlessly" as his words carried her into "another world, completely new and yet strangely familiar and close." She felt herself overcome by emotion and suddenly blurted out, "I must go to India!" (It was only later that Eugenia learned that the book's author, who called himself Yogi Ramacharaka, wasn't actually from India himself. His real name was William Walker Atkinson, and he lived in Chicago.)

Eugenia finally made the journey in her late twenties, and she discovered she adored India in real life even more than she had in her fantasies. "India was to me the land of the fulfillment of my dreams." Unlike most Westerners in the country, she spent most of her time with locals. "I fell in love with the land and its people and made friends with everyone I met," she wrote. She was drawn in by the customs, beliefs, and ways of life of all castes.

What began as a temporary visit turned into an indefinite move to the country. She sold off her fur coats, jewels, and other valuables to get by before finding work as an actress—including a starring role in one of the country's earliest silent films. She adopted an Indian name for the role, appearing in the credits as Indira Devi. Her new surname was Sanskrit for goddess. "She was only one letter away from becoming Indra Devi," writes Goldberg, but "it would take more than another decade to get there."

Amid her budding silent film career, Eugenia met her husband, Jan Strakaty, the Czech commercial attaché to India. They embarked on a high-society life together in Bombay, busy with dinner parties and balls and endless socializing. "Comfortably married, I allowed myself to slip gradually into the whirlpool of society life," she wrote

in 1953. She had traveled to India in search of spiritual enlightenment, but now she found herself in the role of wife and hostess. She
longed for a greater sense of purpose.

"I wasn't actually *doing* anything else," she wrote. "Was this
why I had wanted to come to India? To become a popular hostess and
party-goer? What had happened to my desire to work, to help, to
learn? Something must be done about it, I said to myself. I must
change my life, start all over again."

She had learned a thing or two about yoga during her time in
India, but she had never studied it seriously. Now, feeling buried
alive, she finally sought it out in earnest.

Yoga itself was undergoing a dramatic transformation around this
time, as India's respected civil and spiritual leaders began to consider
its potential as a path to fitness. While ancient yoga texts held that
strengthening the body could allow practitioners to sit and meditate
for longer stretches without being distracted by aches, pains, and
fatigue, over time, yoga as a physical practice had fallen into disre-
pute. "When educated people, whether Indian or Western, spoke respectfully of yoga, they usually meant a system of breathing,
meditation, and philosophy, not physical postures," writes Goldberg.
Physical yoga "was widely seen as the province of magicians, con
men, and sideshow contortionists."

When Eugenia began studying yoga in the 1930s, however, the
leaders of India's independence movement were beginning to
reconsider. Perhaps it was "a superior indigenous type of physical
culture"—a way to build a populace that was physically strong
enough to break free from British control. "This old and typical Indian method of preserving bodily fitness is rather remarkable when
one compares it with the more usual methods involving rushing
about, jerks, hops, and jumps which leave one panting, out of breath,

and tired out," wrote Jawaharlal Nehru, India's future prime minister. Indian yoga gurus strategically combined elements of Western "physical culture," such as bodybuilding and gymnastics, with ancient postures—creating a hybrid practice suited to the needs of their countrymen.

Eugenia's serious yoga training began with a wedding invitation.

She and her husband were friends with the maharaja of Mysore, a city in Southern India, and in 1939, he invited the couple to attend the marriage of his nephew at his palace. Eugenia knew the maharaja to be a progressive leader who was "devoted to spreading the wonders of yoga to the West." He was patron to a very famous yoga guru named Tirumalai Krishnamacharya, who ran a yoga school at the palace.

When Eugenia arrived in Mysore, she went straight to the guru. He told her he had no classes for women, nor foreigners, and asked her to leave. She was disappointed but undeterred and decided to go to Krishnamacharya's boss, the maharaja—who ordered the guru to take on his friend as a disciple.

Krishnamacharya grudgingly put Eugenia on a demanding schedule and ascetic diet. "He was very strict with me, thinking that I would not keep up the regime that he imposed on me," she later said. Eugenia found her new regimen draining at first. In creating his particular brand of yoga, her guru had incorporated "numerous disparate sources, from a twelfth-century text to native gymnastics," writes Stefanie Syman in *The Subtle Body: The Story of Yoga in America*, blending "yogic asanas, elements of Indian wrestling and Western gymnastics, and possibly moves found in British military-training exercises."

Soon, however, Eugenia began to see the results of the program. "Inside of a few months I regained my former girlish figure, wrinkles vanished from my face, and my skin became smooth and firm," she wrote. "In fact everybody commented on my sparkling eyes and my youthful appearance. I felt as light and carefree as a school girl on a summer vacation."

She also earned her guru's respect. "When my teacher saw that I was really serious about my study, he completely changed his attitude towards me," she wrote. "Instead of leaving me to one of his assistants, he started giving me personal instructions, and took a keen interest in my progress."

About a year into her yoga training, the Czech government transferred Eugenia's husband from Bombay to Shanghai. When she told her guru she would need to join him, Krishnamacharya responded that he wanted her to teach yoga in China and wherever else she might travel; he had become convinced, like his patron, that yoga should be spread far and wide. (Krishnamacharya would eventually train B.K.S. Iyengar and K. Pattabhi Jois, who would go on to become the fathers of the extremely popular Iyengar and Ashtanga methods of yoga, respectively. Jois was later accused of sexually abusing his students.)

Eugenia taught what is believed to be the first-ever yoga classes in China, growing her school to more than seventy students, most of whom were the wives of Western diplomats. When Japan seized control of Shanghai during World War II, she convinced authorities to let her teach Brits and Americans interned in prison camps. Finally, when the war ended and Allied forces liberated the city, she returned to Bombay. Her husband returned to Europe, where he would die soon after.

Back in India, Eugenia earned the distinction of being the first Western woman to teach yoga in the country. But when a Chinese general sent a squad of machine gunners to seize control of her house, which he wanted for himself, she felt compelled to return to Shanghai. She sold off her belongings in the city and debated where to go next.

Eventually, she bought boat tickets for both India and California, which friends told her would be fertile ground for her classes. "I decided to leave the matter to the higher power," she said, "resolving to take the boat that would sail first, as there were no regular schedules in those postwar days." The universe revealed: She was bound for Los Angeles.

With her journey west, she shed the last remnants of Eugenia Peterson and became Indra Devi.

When Indra Devi arrived in Los Angeles in early 1947, she landed in a city that was deeply stressed. It was seeing an overwhelming influx of World War II veterans hoping to start a new life in the sun, still grappling with the horrors of war and creating a housing crisis. Violent crime was at an all-time high. And the almighty film industry was rife with suspicion, as the House Committee on Un-American Activities began investigating film artists for communist sympathies—leading to the notorious Hollywood blacklist, which derailed the careers of hundreds and sent a handful to prison.

If anyone could benefit from yoga, Indra Devi thought, it was these people.

Many Angelenos recognized this, too. After the war there was "a great hunger for the insights of the East adapted to address the malaise of the West," writes Goldberg. And yet while a small handful of people offered private yoga lessons in the city, no one was offering the kind of practical, health-focused yoga classes Devi planned to teach—or positioning yoga as a beauty tool.

Devi moved into an apartment housed in a building that had once been a lavish private villa, perched high in the Hollywood Hills, and got to work charming the city's intellectual, artistic, and social elite. She became friends with British novelist turned screenwriter

Aldous Huxley, who happened to be devoted to yoga's spiritual teachings himself, and who granted her access to his rarefied circle of friends.

"She had no job, no family in the country, and no homeland to return to. She was nearing fifty in a city that worshipped ingénues," writes Goldberg. "The only thing left to do," Devi later wrote, "was to begin anew."

She leased a small space on the famed Sunset Strip, just down the street from popular nightclubs. Outside, she planted a wood sign that read INDRA DEVI, YOGA CLASSES, with an arrow pointing to the door.

The space was nearly bare, with sparse white walls displaying a sprinkling of pictures. The floors were covered in cloth mats. Before long, however, her humble studio was attracting everyone from "prominent business managers to little sales girls," she wrote—as well as a who's who of Hollywood movie stars, from Greta Garbo to Gloria Swanson.

Indra Devi became especially close with Swanson, who was an eager disciple. She began teaching the actress shortly after Swanson starred in Billy Wilder's *Sunset Boulevard* as Norma Desmond, a washed-up silent film star obsessed with remaining young and beautiful. Unlike her character, Swanson was flourishing in middle age— hosting a television series, performing on Broadway, and launching a mass-market clothing line called Forever Young. Swanson also remained a beauty icon. A 1951 advertisement for Jergens All-Purpose Cream features the actress's beatific image and asks, "Will you look as young as Gloria Swanson at 51?" Swanson's enthusiasm for yoga helped to boost both Devi's and yoga's popularity.

Devi made it clear: Her studio was not a temple of religion, but one of the body. Friends had advised that for yoga to appeal to Americans—even with their interest in Eastern wisdom—she would have to literally demystify it, and she did. "[She] went to great pains to explain the practice in scientific rather than spiritual terms," writes Goldberg. "Yoga, as she presented it, was first and foremost a commonsense exercise and relaxation system, utterly practical and wholesome, promising transformative results without the grunting agony of other physical culture regimens."

Devi taught in flowing shorts and sleeveless shirts, while her students dressed mostly in leotards and stockings. Her Russian accent made her sound something like a ballet instructor. "As a teacher, Devi was both gracious and exacting," writes Syman. She began classes with simple breathing exercises, before guiding her students through postures. "The experience was gentle and even relaxing. Her students didn't sweat profusely . . . or hold poses until their muscles quivered. No, Devi insisted that to strain was to defeat the purpose."

As Indra Devi's fame grew, so did the opportunities to speak publicly about yoga as exercise—a concept that was still foreign to most women. After a presentation before a Los Angeles chapter of Eaters Anonymous, a woman in the front row asked her, "How often do you take yogurt?" Taken aback, Devi answered, "Well, I couldn't say exactly; sometimes every day, sometimes not." Then Devi had a realization: "You don't think, by any chance, that I was lecturing on *yogurt* tonight?" she asked. *Why yes*, the woman responded, she did.

On the East Coast, cosmetics mogul and spa owner Elizabeth Arden had sworn by the salubrious benefits of yoga for years—she would often position herself in a handstand inside her famous Red Door Spa in New York City as aestheticians beautified society women. In 1950, she invited Devi to teach at her exclusive Maine Chance health and beauty retreats in Maine and Arizona—rustic "camps" where wealthy ladies would go on restrictive diets and take in the great outdoors. Devi was a hit at the retreats, helping to position yoga into even more of an acceptable bourgeois hobby. Arden later flew Devi to New York for private lessons. "She wanted me to join her staff," Devi told *Yoga Journal* in 1996, but she refused. "I would not work for anyone."

Indra Devi was living a fairy tale. There was just one hitch: The U.S. government had received an anonymous letter claiming Devi was actually a Soviet spy. "Under the 'veil' of yoga," the tipster claimed, she had "penetrated everywhere." Now the FBI was on her case.

When federal agents interviewed Devi's friends and acquaintances, they all called the charge "absurd." Most suspected the tip came from the wife of a man who had become enamored of Devi in China. Still, this was the height of the McCarthy era, and suspected commies were guilty until proven innocent. "Devi was a Russian with multiple aliases and a suspiciously bohemian lifestyle," writes Goldberg. When FBI agents told director J. Edgar Hoover they had found nothing suspicious, he told them to "look harder." It would take nearly a decade for Devi to shake the charges and become an American citizen.

The big break that would make Indra Devi a household name came from a self-help book. As her profile grew, the publisher Prentice Hall offered Devi a deal, and in 1953 she published *Forever Young, Forever Healthy*. Gloria Swanson suggested the title, inspired by her clothing line, and provided a blurb for the cover. The book also advertised endorsements from actress Linda Christian, the first Bond girl (in a TV adaptation of *Casino Royale*), and modern dance pioneer Ruth St. Denis, teacher to legendary choreographer Martha Graham.

Forever Young, Forever Healthy opens with Devi's personal story of salvation through yoga, before offering a straightforward guide to improving one's health, mood, and physical appearance.

"This book is written with only one purpose in mind: to share with you the remarkable experiences I have undergone," Devi writes in the foreword, "experiences which transformed me from a sick, nervous and unhappy woman into a happy human being, healthy and relaxed both physically and mentally."

Her book promises to help readers address everything from headaches to fatigue to constipation, as well as relief from "stress"—a term popularized in the fifties. Many of her students were plagued by "nerves" or a diffuse malaise, feelings she knew all too well. She offered up yoga as an alternative to the tranquilizers that became so popular throughout the decade. Devi is also strikingly candid about sex, declaring that men are responsible for satisfying their wives' erotic desires. And she is enlightened in her thinking about women's rights, writing that women will suffer "until man grants woman equality as a human being."

But despite Devi's progressive views, she also included a chapter titled "The Woman Beautiful," in which she asks readers: "Are you as beautiful as you can be?" She goes on to instruct them in the same rather brutal manner as Bonnie Prudden did: Women should stand naked before a full-length mirror and examine their body from head to toe. "Is there anything you don't like about it? Your hips perhaps? Or your stomach?" Whatever so-called figure faults they spot, she continues, are *their* fault. "Is it because you take too many drinks, or eat too much or smoke too much? Perhaps you are too fond of sweets and pastries. Or perhaps you are too lazy and do not exercise enough. . . . If it's exercise you need do not say that you have no time for it. If a busy person like Elizabeth Arden, for instance, the busiest woman I have ever known, finds time for exercising, there is no reason why anyone else cannot do the same." The book is sprinkled with photos of conventionally attractive, smiling young women in leotards, demonstrating various postures. None appear to be straining or sweating.

Devi herself wore no makeup or girdles or high-heeled shoes. But she was very trim. She justified her focus on helping women transform their appearance by highlighting yoga's spiritual teachings about the body. Yogis, she writes, "keep the body healthy, beautiful, shapely and clean, within and without, because they regard it as a vehicle through which the Supreme Power manifests itself. To them the body is a temple of the Living Spirit and, therefore, they believe in bringing it to the highest state of perfection."

Devi's publisher sent her on a cross-country publicity tour, and *Forever Young, Forever Healthy* became a national bestseller. She spoke at women's clubs, health conferences, and spiritual centers, and she appeared on television at least twice. The book would soon catch on internationally, too, as it was translated into French, German, Spanish, Portuguese, and Italian.

After the success of *Forever Young, Forever Healthy*, Prentice Hall commissioned Devi to write two more books. In 1959, she published *Yoga for Americans*, which offered a more detailed, prescriptive guide to her yoga exercises. Along the way, she met and married her second husband—a German doctor named Sigfrid Knauer, who specialized in natural (if not exactly scientifically sound) medicine. She was thriving.

Around 1960, Devi and her husband relocated to Tecate, Mexico—she had fallen in love with the country while visiting a wealthy friend who owned a large villa. When her friend died, she purchased the villa herself, which happened to be next door to the world-famous health spa Rancho La Puerta—co-owned by the same woman who owned the Golden Door Spa in San Diego, the same woman who would hire Judi Sheppard Missett and Tamilee Webb early in their careers. The spa owners were early adopters of most modern exercise programs, and they loved the idea of working with a yoga teacher. They convinced Devi to turn her new home into a yoga school for spa-goers.

One of Devi's Rancho La Puerta clients was the founder and owner of a clothing company that produced the country's first line of stylish maternity clothes—a company called Page Boy, based in Dallas, Texas. This woman was so enthusiastic about Indra Devi and yoga that she invited her to visit her factory and teach yoga to her employees on the factory floor.

In November 1963, Devi flew to Dallas for the training. When she learned that President John F. Kennedy would be in the city at the same time, she wanted to meet him and hoped to "teach him some deep-breathing exercises that he might use to cope with the enormous strain of his job," writes Goldberg.

But Kennedy was assassinated before she had the opportunity.

Devi was deeply shaken by the president's death—so much so that it inspired her to travel to Vietnam in 1966, at the height of the Vietnam War, five years before Jane Fonda would make her own pilgrimage to the country. She hoped she might spread peace and love through yogic meditations. "She doesn't seem to have had a plan in place for what would happen when she got there," writes Goldberg, "but she was used to charging into the unknown and having it work out."

But she didn't stay long. Despite yoga's transformative power, she saw upon her arrival that her regimen couldn't, in fact, end that horrific war.

Back in America, however, Indra Devi's impact was undeniable: Thanks to her savvy and tireless promotion of yoga, the practice was helping scores of middle- and upper-class white women navigate mental and emotional challenges. Still, it would be decades before yoga would become the cultural behemoth that it is today.

Throughout the sixties, Middle America gradually began to consider yoga an acceptable path to physical fitness—despite the fact that the country's brewing counterculture was also turning to yoga for more far-out purposes. In 1965, President Lyndon Johnson ended a nearly fifty-year quota system for immigrants from India, which led waves of Indian yoga masters to bring their methods to America. Counterculture icons from renegade Harvard psychologist Timothy Leary to poet Allen Ginsberg raved about yoga's power to create harmony with the universe, particularly when practiced while dropping acid. At the same time, however, perfectly square Americans gradually took it up to unwind from the stresses of the office and raising kids—and to achieve lithe and limber bodies.

In January 1961, the *Los Angeles Times* launched a twelve-part series in its Family Section under the headline "Yoga for All." The first article began: "Everybody's talking about yoga. But just what is it? Do you have to be a beatnik to enjoy it? Won't you feel pretty silly sitting in a full lotus position, practicing oriental mediation [sic]?"

The article's author continues: Yoga isn't a "strange rite practiced by an oddball religious sect" but "combinations of body exercises, breathing practices, diets and concentration exercises which devoted yogis swear beat a barrelful of 20th century 'calm down' or 'wake up' pills."

That same year, as part of what *Sponsor* magazine dubbed "TV's Great Bust-and-Chest Boom," Los Angeles's KTTV began broadcasting a program called *Yoga for Health*. The series was hosted by a yoga teacher named Richard Hittleman. Within a year it went national.

Hittleman was born to Jewish parents in the Bronx, but as a young man, he found himself pulled toward Zen Buddhism. In August 1961 he told *The Washington Post*, "I was first introduced to yoga as a kid by an East Indian who worked as a dishwasher at [my] parents' hotel in the Adirondacks. . . . He was my guru . . . and since he showed me how it was done I've never looked back." (If you were looking for an on-the-nose example of why yoga as practiced by

Americans has been accused of cultural appropriation—well, there you go.)

Hittleman moved to Hollywood in his early thirties and sold TV execs on his idea for a series, which led viewers through basic yoga poses, spicing up "knee bends and torso twists with zestful talk on diet and gentle reprimands." Soon his audience grew to include "housewives, business executives and movie stars who [joined] him daily." His assistant on the show was a woman named Diane Stewart, who appeared in full makeup, coiffed hair, and tight-fitting catsuits—or, as the *Post* put it, "a shapely young lady who gives the men something to look at while the ladies are listening to Hittleman."

The host said he received some six hundred letters a week from viewers.

Hittleman apparently saw his series as a solution to mid-century women's problems. "American women are a mess," he told the *Post*. "They're falling apart. They suffer from advanced gadgetitis." (Yes, that's definitely the main reason women in the early sixties were suffering, Richard.) He would go on to write several bestselling yoga books, geared primarily toward these sad specimens of womanhood.*

Meanwhile, women's magazines sold yoga as an "ancient beauty secret." In 1965, *Cosmopolitan* ran a feature headlined "How Yoga Can Change Your Life." *Seventeen* pitched it as a healthy regimen for teen girls. "Models do it—because it's good for the figure," one feature began. "Dancers do it—because it helps keep them supple." By 1968, even the Beatles were doing it, albeit more for transcendence than to firm up their midsections—though the band's

---

* Hittleman's first book, *Yoga: 28 Day Exercise Plan,* was Workman Publishing's first-ever title. Nearly two decades later, this same house would publish Tamilee Webb's *Rubber Band Workout.*

endorsement surely convinced some young fans to give it a go. For women who wanted more personal instruction, yoga was increasingly offered at YWCAs.

In 1969, Hittleman opened up a yoga school in a former banquet hall above New York City's Grand Central Station, where he taught office workers and housewives as commuter trains and subways whizzed beneath them. By the end of the sixties, "yoga was something the hippies had in common with their putative enemies: the middle-class conformist, the corporate drone, the happy housewife," writes Stefanie Syman. "The discipline was to grow hugely among both groups."

Feminist leaders embraced yoga as part of their push for women's physical autonomy. Women's consciousness-raising groups incorporated yoga into their meetings, and in 1971, the authors of *Our Bodies, Ourselves* recommended it to readers. "Yoga is not just for Eastern mystics and American hippies," they write. "In our tense and aggressive society, yoga's total lack of competitiveness is a wonderful release."

———————————

But even greater numbers of women, including those who had never ventured near a consciousness-raising group, discovered yoga through a fresh-faced TV host who *Time* billed as the "Julia Child of Yoga."

Three times a week, Lilias Folan—the mother of two young boys in Cincinnati, Ohio—led viewers through asanas on a popular PBS series called *Lilias, Yoga and You*, picking up the proverbial baton from Indra Devi to become, for many years, the country's most visible female teacher of yoga.

Lilias, Yoga and You aired right before *Sesame Street*, and many moms caught it unintentionally. Flipping on the TV for their kids, they would find Lilias, sheathed in a pink bodysuit. She wore her thick brown hair in a long braid. She appeared every bit the pretty "girl next door."

Early episodes of *Lilias, Yoga and You* feel something like *Mister Rogers' Neighborhood* for grown women. Lilias appears alone on the screen and speaks directly to the camera in calm, reassuring tones, encouraging women to reflect on their lives without judgment. From the beginning, she tried to speak into the camera as if she was speaking to a friend, she told me in an interview.

"Hello, class. Namaste. Hello, and how are you today?" she says at the top of a 1974 episode. "You don't necessarily have to be terribly happy even to come to class, but as long as you're here, that's marvelous. You know, I think I'm very much a realist about life and living—especially in my own life, too—that there are peaks and that there are valleys, and that this is really very much how our life goes." From there, she reflects on yoga's ability to nurture mental health as well as physical health.

The series "introduced so many women to something that was [still] considered really spooky and abnormal and weird," Lilias told me, assuring them "it was none of those things."

Lilias had discovered yoga in the mid-sixties, at an emotional low point in her life. She was in her late twenties, and she spent her days as a housewife and mother in Darien, Connecticut, weighed down by fatigue and depression. Her family doctor told her there was nothing wrong with her physically, but that she might consider exercise—a progressive recommendation at the time. She decided to try yoga.

"I put myself in the back row of one of the first yoga classes [in New York City], and I really enjoyed it," she told me. With time, she began to notice physical changes—she was more flexible than she'd been since childhood—but the more profound changes were internal. She felt calmer and slept more soundly.

Lilias and her family then moved to Cincinnati, where she

taught yoga classes herself at a YWCA. The TV series came about thanks to one of her students, who was married to a producer for the local public broadcasting channel. The student told her husband: "This is something that should be televised, and I've got the perfect person to teach it."

Lilias, Yoga and You first aired locally in 1970, and it was a hit. She went on to write a book by the same name, which also took off locally—it was even translated into braille so blind readers could follow along. The book covered yoga basics and offered advice on diet, the power of positive thinking, and yoga as a tool for physical transformation. "If you want a beautiful or handsome body, you will have it with Hatha Yoga," Lilias writes. (*Hatha yoga* is the term for the physical practice of yoga.) "What you put into these exercises you will get back, doubled!" But, crucially, she veers from Devi: "I am really 'bugged' with fashion magazines that constantly encourage youthfulness, for men and women, as a goal in life. How absurd!" Instead, she advises, consider yoga a path to cultivating contentment and balance as one ages.

In 1974, *Lilias, Yoga and You* went national on PBS, where it aired for twenty-five years. "Looking back," she told me, "I believe it was something I was put on the planet to do."

There was one thing that made Lilias self-conscious: sweating on camera. She had been taught that women weren't supposed to sweat, and she would surreptitiously dab her forehead with a towel. "You know, 'nice women don't sweat,'" she told me. This was a challenge, given the bright studio lights.

(She apparently pulled it off, at least in the eyes of one male newspaper columnist. In 1979, the *San Francisco Chronicle*'s Gerald Nachman declared: "I've fallen head over heels for the television yoga lady . . . By far her most intriguing aspect is that she never sweats." He goes on to explain: "Of course, I've always been a push-over for exercise ladies, on TV or in cold print, and I still wonder whatever became of that alluring tease, Bonnie Prudden, who pushed her way up from obscurity in the back pages of *Sports Illustrated* during my fevered teenage years." Thank you for sharing, Gerald.)

Lilias received bags of letters from viewers, detailing how her series had changed their lives. The series also had a profound effect on some of her youngest viewers. My friend Jessica remembers watching Lilias as a seven-year-old on Long Island, New York, noting how the calm vibe she projected was so different from her own tumultuous home life; Jessica went on to become a yoga teacher herself. On an archival video channel for Lilias's series, one woman commented: "I first saw *Lilias, Yoga and You* when I was twelve . . . Living alone with my Mother, who lived with schizophrenia—I found this program, this woman, comforting. Lilias, with her soothing reassuring voice and different type of exercises, were indeed my refuge."

In 1975, the year after *Lilias, Yoga and You* went national, a group of yoga devotees in San Francisco launched the publication that would become *Yoga Journal*, helping to create a national community for the country's yoga instructors. "This was the missing media link," writes Stefanie Syman, "a publication by insiders that, like *Runner's World* or *Popular Mechanics*, would give this subculture a voice but not limit itself to a single teacher or technique."

The seventies also saw the rise of modern yoga mats. In 1967, the British yoga pioneer Angela Farmer forgot her mat for a class she was teaching in Germany and grabbed a piece of foam carpet padding to use instead. Until then, most yogis practiced on towels or cotton cloths, which could slip on smooth surfaces. Back in London, Farmer began offering the nonslip padding to students, who preferred it to cloth, and together with her father, she began mass producing the first "sticky" mats.

But as the eighties got under way, aerobics, weight training, and gym culture overshadowed yoga. After decades of growth, the percentage of Americans who practiced began to decrease. "Aerobics emphasized power and strength, as women climbed career ladders and started competing more directly with men in much greater numbers," writes Syman. "Its benefits were, in a word, masculine. To practice yoga was to move slowly and deliberately, being careful not to strain or overexert yourself. Yoga was gentle, relaxing, and safe, qualities not likely to help you break through the glass ceiling."

There were a few notable exceptions, however, that would prove key for yoga's eventual explosion. In the seventies, an instructor named Bikram Choudhury arrived in Beverly Hills from India and began teaching yoga in a room that was intentionally hot, to intensify the workout. His approach was more drill sergeant than loving guide, and his classes grew to include the city's power elite. He began calling himself "Yogi to the Stars," and as his empire expanded, he bought himself a collection of Rolls-Royces.

In 1984, *Sports Illustrated* sat in on one of his classes, held in the mezzanine of a high-rise on Wilshire Boulevard. "There are about two dozen men and women stretching and sweating," the reporter notes, while Choudhury—who taught in a Speedo and a Rolex watch, his hair pulled back into a ponytail—"sits on blue satin cushions at the front of the room and abuses his well-heeled clientele: 'You have money! You come to me for pain, you Beverly Heels people! You pay me to hurt you!'"

Bikram Choudhury would spawn a national trend of what was previously called Bikram Yoga. It has since been renamed hot yoga, however, after several women accused its founder of rape and sexual assault, as well as false imprisonment, discrimination, and sexual harassment, leading him to be called the "Harvey Weinstein of Yoga."

Yoga evolved in less controversial ways throughout the eighties, too.

In 1984, a progressive husband-and-wife team opened the Jivamukti yoga center in Manhattan's East Village, where they infused yoga with a spirit of rock and roll. They offered physically intense classes set to contemporary music, and the center would grow into a celebrity hot spot. In 1984, actress and high-intensity-crotch-leotard icon Raquel Welch published *Raquel: The Raquel Welch Total Beauty and Fitness Program*, which featured hatha yoga as its core exercise regimen.

Gradually, the yoga that was practiced in the shadow of the gym boom became more athletic, more steeped in the language of fitness culture—evolving to meet women where they were at the dawn of the next decade.

―――――――――

The nineties is when yoga truly went mainstream. While women had more rights than their mothers did a generation ago, they also faced unprecedented challenges. Sure, *technically*, they could strive for nearly any job they wanted and also be a wife and mother . . . but they earned less money than men in the same careers. No public support existed to *help* working mothers "have it all"—no universal maternity leave policy, no childcare, nothing. Women were stressed like never before, and popular culture suggested it was all *their* fault—for daring to want lives outside the home, for cultivating professional ambition as well as personal ambition. *You asked for this*, pundits said. *Are you happy now?*

Against this backdrop, the nineties would see what author Allison Yarrow calls the "bitchification" of public figures, as high-powered women who threatened the status quo or appeared a little *too* confident in their power were publicly punished. Hillary Clinton, Anita Hill, Monica Lewinsky—they all became cultural villains, fair game for ridicule and mockery.

It's no wonder women of the nineties gravitated toward a

workout that promised sanctuary, affirmation, and inner peace. After all, as yogis told their students, yoga's most recognizable symbol,
the lotus flower, begins its life in muddy water before bursting
through the surface and blossoming.

Throughout the decade, the fitness world began to embrace yoga
with unprecedented enthusiasm, as the number of American women
who practiced ballooned by tens of millions. Yoga studios began popping up in strip malls across America. Gyms began adding yoga to
their class offerings. New, increasingly athletic varieties of yoga
emerged, including power yoga.

Then came the celebrities. Madonna became an especially enthusiastic proponent of yoga—she even included a Sanskrit chant in her
1998 album *Ray of Light.* "It's the '90s and the woman appears more
spiritual than material," observed a writer for *Yoga Journal.* "Again,
she is right on the zeitgeist: after all, she is Madonna." *The New York
Times* declared, "The yoga body—loose-jointed and lean-muscled—
is this year's look." Also in 1998, Oprah demonstrated asanas on her
show. Yoga had arrived.

By 2001, *Time*'s Richard Corliss reported: "Yoga now straddles
the continent—from Hollywood, where $20 million-a-picture actors
queue for a session with their guru du jour, to Washington, where,
in the gym of the Supreme Court, Justice Sandra Day O'Connor and
15 others faithfully take their class each Tuesday morning."

The more Americans practiced yoga, however, the more yoga culture began to reinforce some of the very same pressures women were
trying to escape. It became increasingly focused on achievement and
on outward appearances. Some classes began to feel competitive.

"Like any other force, the power and energy cultivated through
yoga can be used to buttress the ego and fuel narcissism," warned a
Yoga Journal article in 1998. "Everyone knows someone (not us, of
course) whose arrogance has only increased as their back bends have
deepened. As media feeds us images of yoga at its most superficial,

it's important to remember its deepest purpose—to still the mind and open the heart."

America had long since embraced the notion that a fit body was a virtuous body. Now, with yoga's focus on "bringing it to the highest state of perfection," as Indra Devi had described it, the cultural imperative to work out became even more explicit. Meanwhile, as Americans' involvement with organized religion continued to decline, yoga rose to fill many women's spiritual needs.

By the late nineties, yoga was billed as the exercise of supermodels, from Christy Turlington to Shalom Harlow—creating the impression that it was an activity for the already thin, privileged, and beautiful. In her 1998 feature for *Yoga Journal* on yoga's startling transformation into something "chic," Anne Cushman notes: "Sure, we've been saying for years that everyone should do this, but now that everyone really is, we fret that the true practice—like everything from filmmaking to yogurt—is being Nutra-sweetened and dumbed down to suit the tastes of the American mass market."

Yoga Journal co-founder Judith Lasater put it this way: "Our culture doesn't honor just being present, but instead we honor doing, productivity, and action. And so where do we go now for rest and recuperation?"

Yoga became a major industry and capitalist force, something longtime yogis found troubling, given the practice's focus on aspiring to spiritual over material wealth. "Where there's a yoga blitz, there must be yoga biz," Corliss wrote in *Time*. "To dress for a class, you need only some old, loose-fitting clothes—and since you perform barefoot, no fancy footwear." And yet, Nike and J.Crew and even Christy Turlington had developed yoga apparel, he noted. "For those who prefer stay-at-home yoga, the video-store racks groan with hot, moving tapes." Yoga-wear behemoth Lululemon was founded in 1998, as body-hugging yoga pants became the new leotards.

Beyond workout gear, yoga was used to sell everything "from soft drinks to designer evening wear, somehow suggesting that 'if you acquired the right things, you'll be happy,'" writes Cushman. This was "a delusion that real yogis have worked for centuries to undo." Not only that, she mourns, there's the "subliminal message contained in these messages: that yoga is about looking good, and that if you just do enough Sun Salutations, you won't have to grow old and die."

Of course, millions of women did find the solace and strength they were looking for in yoga, despite its complexities—numbers that have continued to grow. Today the global yoga industry is valued at more than $37 billion.

———————————

In recent years, yoga's popularity among thin white middle- and upper-class women, in particular, has sparked an important and overdue conversation about who has been excluded from yoga, as well as yoga's troubling legacy as a form of cultural appropriation.

"Those without access to an in-depth history education might lighten this to a question of political correctness or cries by minorities for cultural recognition. But it goes so much deeper," Rina Deshpande, a first-generation Indian American yoga researcher and teacher, wrote in *Yoga Journal* in 2019. "Today, yoga is often marketed by affluent Westerners to affluent Westerners—and Indians, ironically, are marginally represented, if at all. While this multibillion-dollar industry is offering much-needed well-being to Western practitioners, it's re-inflicting the same violation on India and Indians: invisibility and misrepresentation."

For Deshpande and so many other South Asian yoga disciples, this cultural whitewashing feels profoundly personal. "I often ponder why this means so much to me and why I can't offer simple bullet points for what makes something 'appreciative' versus 'appropriative' of yoga," she writes. "I just know when I start to feel sick or hurt." Such as when yoga business owners have suggested to her that incorporating any Eastern elements into a class "will threaten the comfort of white American practitioners." Or, alternately, "when I'm walking by a shop with my parents, only to see their confusion over why holy Hindu scriptures—which my father can read, being literate in Sanskrit—were printed on a hoodie and tossed into a sale pile."

Rina Deshpande's voice is one of a growing chorus calling for greater awareness of the way yoga is practiced by Westerners. This cultural reeducation is still in its very early stages, but the fact that there is now a very public dialogue around yoga as a form of appropriation—in traditional and social media, among the leadership of yoga businesses and classes—offers signs of progress.

I spoke with PBS's Lilias Folan on a snowy Thursday morning in February 2021. I was ensconced in my apartment, surrounded by dusty copies of Indra Devi's books and piles of thirty-year-old issues of *Shape*. Lilias, then eighty-four years old and a grandmother of seven, was sipping coffee in her home in Cincinnati.

We were nearing the one-year anniversary of the coronavirus lockdown, around the time articles started popping up about hitting the pandemic "wall." Social media had devolved into a heated debate over whether women should part their hair to the side or down the middle—and whether the former marked a woman as "old."

On that particular day, as I smoothed my side part, I felt what so many mothers had described to me before I became one myself—a feeling of being pulled between the demands of work and parenthood and not entirely succeeding at either. This, despite having a supportive and involved husband and every creature comfort. Some writing deadlines had been missed and others were looming, so screen time in our home had ballooned from minutes to hours—and I had recently acquiesced to my toddler's request for cookies for breakfast.

Lilias and I spoke about her career and life and yoga practice. As we were wrapping up, she said in a singsongy voice, "Remember to remember to exhale, Danielle!"

I felt my eyes well up with tears.

Her comment, which felt so personal in that moment, had caught me off guard. I felt embarrassed by my emotional overflow, brought on by something she probably says to everyone. But I also felt a weight lift from my shoulders. Suddenly I got it. *So this is why women like yoga.*

I told her I would try to remember. She said *namaste.*

Today, at a time of unprecedented social and cultural stress, yoga is practiced by more than 36 million Americans, 70 percent of whom are women. But the *promise* of yoga—that exercise can offer a salve not only for the body but also for the soul, that fitness studios can be places of transcendence—has become even more culturally pervasive. When SoulCycle promises a kind of religious experience via stationary bike, when barre studios display sidewalk signs telling women to "believe," they are channeling the hope of the yoga boom of the late twentieth century.

When I spoke with Judith Lasater, the co-founding editor of *Yoga Journal* who has been teaching yoga for five decades, she told me this: "Women are longing—*longing*—for refuge. Sometimes refuge can be a long run by yourself. Sometimes it can just be lying on a mat." Sometimes a boutique fitness studio can provide it.

But she cautioned, "refuge is an intention, not a location." And it doesn't come from executing a perfect forward bend. More often than not, she told me, refuge comes simply from showing ourselves a little kindness.

CHAPTER 8

Expand

We are not meant to be perfect; we are meant to be whole.

—Jane Fonda

To be rather than to seem.

—State motto of North Carolina, tattooed
in Latin on Jessamyn Stanley's right arm

When I run through my neighborhood on New York's Upper East Side, sheathed in high-tech Lycra blends, I am surrounded by women in motion. When I first started writing this book, the streets hummed with women coming and going from gyms and boutique fitness studios. Through the coronavirus pandemic, they masked up to jog, tuck, lift, dance, stretch, and walk in Central Park, keenly aware of how vital movement was to their mental and emotional health. In this city, where private lives are lived so publicly, I sometimes spot women through building windows spinning on stationary bikes in their living rooms. Heart-pumping, sweat-inducing exercise, once an affront to conventional notions of femininity, is now a defining ritual of upper-middle-class womanhood.

The past twenty years have brought women a dazzling array of fitness offerings. With the rise of yoga, women were reminded that the physical space in which they care for their body doesn't have to be a sprawling multiplex of sizzling spandex—it can just be a small, simple studio with an intimate gathering of women. This realization helped fuel the explosion of boutique fitness studios. Pilates, the stretching and strengthening workout invented by German strong man Joseph Pilates during World War I, soared in this country alongside yoga. The Bar Method and Pure Barre were both founded in 2001. SoulCycle was founded in 2006 and cross-training franchise Orangetheory in 2010. Over the next decade, boutique brands would multiply to become the fixtures they are today. They would also inspire dozens of spin-offs and hybrids—offering boxing and rowing and boot camps and cardio dance and every combination in between.

The coronavirus lockdown rocked the fitness industry, as brick-and-mortar gyms and studios were forced to close or drastically limit the number of exercisers allowed inside at a given time. With soaring unemployment and other financial turmoil, fewer people had the resources to spend on fitness. But it also fueled remarkable innovations, as franchises from Jazzercise to Pure Barre moved their classes online, personal trainers offered Zoom sessions, and road races became virtual. Peloton, the at-home fitness brand and subscription service, saw record sales of bikes and treadmills. During a time of unprecedented collective vulnerability, the opportunity to be physically active provided many women with an indispensable form of self-care.

Since Bonnie Prudden began studying the effects of physical activity (and inactivity) seventy years ago, we now have a massive body of scientific research confirming the astounding impact exercise can have on our health and well-being. Regular exercise improves brain health, reducing depression and anxiety. It keeps us mentally sharp as we age. It helps us sleep more soundly. It lowers the risk for heart disease, diabetes, and some cancers. And it strengthens bones and (of course) muscles, which makes navigating everyday life easier.

Regular physical activity is also correlated with a greater sense of purpose in life. As psychologist Kelly McGonigal writes in *The Joy of Movement*: "Movement is intertwined with some of the most basic human joys, including self-expression, social connection, and mastery." Scientists recently discovered that when we exercise, beyond a simple "endorphin high," our bodies produce chemicals that foster hope, empathy, and courage. "When physical activity is most psychologically fulfilling," she continues, "it's because our participation both reveals the good in us and lets us witness the good in others."

But my Upper East Side enclave of exercise devotees tells only part of the story of women's fitness history, offering a skewed view of the movement's success. Despite everything we now know about the benefits of physical activity, having the time, space, and means to exercise remains a privilege. Only a quarter of Americans meet the Centers for Disease Control and Prevention's aerobic and muscle-strengthening exercise recommendations, and just over half even meet the recommended requirements for daily physical activity.

Over the past two decades, fitness has increasingly been sold as a luxury good. In 2019, Americans paid more than ever to work out, between $50 and $150 a month. (For women paying the now-standard boutique fitness fee of $35 per class, that figure was more like $150 per *week*.)

But exercise does not need to be expensive. "The opportunity to engage in physical activity that enables a healthy life should not be a privilege or choice, but a right," argues the Global Wellness Institute, a nonprofit research and advocacy group. And yet, "as the fitness industry develops more and more choices for those who are able and can afford to exercise, there remains a massive swath of inactive population who have limited options." People who live in low-income, rural, and other marginalized communities have significantly less access to fitness facilities and instruction—despite the fact that these communities are at higher risk of chronic disease and could arguably benefit from exercise the most.

For people who *do* have the access and income to work out, the contemporary understanding of what fitness means is often a barrier. After the collective burnout of the early nineties, America's mindset shifted once again, thanks largely to millennials (you're welcome)—a generation conditioned to prioritize productivity and achievement at almost any cost. The millennial-driven fitness industry often positions exercise as a kind of second job, in which we should "optimize" our workouts and forever strive to go faster and harder while meticulously tracking the results. As historian Shelly McKenzie observes, "The formalization of exercise as a practice—a process that has taken place mainly through the lens of consumer culture—has made us much more serious about our exercise routines and, I would argue, has removed at least some of the pleasure from physical activity."

To be sure, challenging yourself to become stronger and achieving a previously out-of-reach goal can be tremendously fulfilling, particularly for women. But this cultural mindset also perpetuates the idea that in order to be active, you have to commit to a rigorous, time-consuming new lifestyle. (The messaging isn't subtle. One needs only to walk by an Equinox and see the tagline IT'S NOT FITNESS. IT'S LIFE scrawled in huge letters in the window to get the idea.)

"To most people, exercising requires substantial overhead: special clothing, a lengthy block of time, and a designated workout space," notes McKenzie. "In the absence of any of these factors, people often choose to do nothing—when, in fact, a twenty-minute walk around the block would have been a healthy choice."

Despite the social progress of the past seven decades, women still face additional obstacles. The fitness industry's focus on aesthetic transformation and weight loss—its glorification of a thin, conventionally feminine ideal—has led too many women to feel deeply uncomfortable in gyms and studios. And the industry's overwhelming whiteness and heteronormativity has led many to feel that they don't belong. It's tough to feel physically free, let alone powerful, in an environment where you are the only person of color or fat person* or gender nonconforming person in the room.

And yet when future historians write about this era of fitness, they may record it as the moment when all of this finally began to change. Over the past few years, a new generation of fitness pioneers has been working to ensure that *all* women have the tools to feel proud of their bodies, to feel strong, and to feel the joy of movement. They are working to challenge assumptions of what a "fit body" looks like. They are working to make exercise about acceptance, not aesthetic transformation, and to make it affordable and accessible for everyone. If the rise of women's fitness represents the fruits of second-wave feminists, the next chapter in fitness history promises to be one that reflects the ideals of third- and fourth-wave feminists: smashing persistent gender norms, acknowledging intersectionality, and honoring the experiences and traumas of marginalized women.

In the previous century, female fitness pioneers succeeded by pushing social boundaries while still playing by conventional rules, stealthily convincing a patriarchal society to accept women's

---

* Within the body-acceptance movement—and in particular, among the activists featured in this chapter—*fat* is the preferred terminology. For this reason, I have chosen to use it in this chapter. Activists point out that *overweight* suggests all humans should strive to be one uniform weight, and *obese* unjustly pathologizes large bodies.

physical empowerment by selling it as a beauty tool. But a vanguard of women's fitness leaders is saying enough is enough. Forget conventions: Why play by the rules when the rules have only held you back?

The twenty-first-century fitness revolution is embodied by Jessamyn Stanley, one of the contemporary industry's most sought-after superstars. For the past decade, Jessamyn—a yoga guru who is Black, queer, femme, and fat—has been offering up herself as evidence that true physical empowerment comes not from transforming yourself to meet our culture's narrow vision of beauty but from self-acceptance. She is, as *Yoga Journal* put it, a "one-woman visibility crusader" for body diversity and inclusion, working to inspire those who have been underserved by mainstream fitness. When she appeared on the cover of that magazine, the headline for her feature read: "Burning Down the House."

Jessamyn Stanley's story began, as so many stories do today, on Instagram.

For most of modern American history, women's magazines, advertisers, and celebrities had a virtual monopoly on dictating women's body ideals: These cultural power brokers told women how to look, and women attempted to abide. It was, for the most part, a one-way conversation.

But with the rise of Instagram and Twitter throughout the 2010s, that paradigm began to shift. For the first time, women had a very public forum in which to respond—and to promote alternative visions. They had "authorship of how we were seen," body-acceptance activist Virgie Tovar told me in a 2019 interview. "Social media has created a voice for the people who have always been the majority in number but not in influence."

With innovation comes an inevitable trade-off—Instagram also perpetuates unrealistic and often toxic beauty standards, and the platform abounds with self-proclaimed fitness experts whose only qualification is their lack of visible body fat. But Jessamyn Stanley and other body-acceptance advocates agree that its power to create a voice for the voiceless, to make previously invisible lifestyles visible, cannot be overstated.

If it weren't for Instagram, Jessamyn wouldn't have risen to fitness icon status. She wouldn't have graced the covers of major magazines, starred in U by Kotex tampon commercials, or been featured on just about every lifestyle television program. She might not even have stuck with yoga. Before she logged onto Instagram, "I was practicing yoga at home, and it was really isolating," she told me in an interview. "There is incredible community to be found on social media."

Growing up in a working-class home outside Greensboro, North Carolina, Jessamyn had a keen sense from a young age that she didn't belong. In elementary school, she wanted to be petite and blond; instead, she had a "wide nose, big belly, big ass, big lips, dark skin."

As she wrote in her 2017 book, *Every Body Yoga: Let Go of Fear, Get On the Mat, Love Your Body,* by the end of fourth grade, "I'd sustained enough failed puppy love crushes on my Jonathan Taylor Thomas–inspired male classmates to realize I didn't really fit into the traditional definition of pretty. Thanks to my subscriptions to *Teen* and *Seventeen* (which I read religiously and held in the absolute highest esteem) I was very familiar with society's agreed-upon vision of beauty. And, as much as it pained me to admit it, I knew for sure that the accepted image didn't have jack shit to do with me."

Jessamyn's dad was an amateur bodybuilder when he was young, and he swore by Pilates. (He still does.) The stretching helped to soothe his muscles, which were often knotted from driving a UPS truck for long hauls—one of two jobs he worked to support their family. But throughout her childhood, Jessamyn saw herself as hopelessly nonathletic and uncoordinated, and she looked for every excuse to get out of PE class.

Only one physical activity interested her: As a middle schooler inspired by the cult film *Bring It On*, she desperately wanted to be a cheerleader—the ultimate marker of social acceptance. But she struggled to make it through the warm-up at tryouts.

As a preteen, she entered a local beauty pageant and, thanks to her beaming smile and infectious charm, she was crowned first runner-up. This earned her a ticket to a national pageant in Orlando, Florida—where she was immediately eliminated in the first round of judging. "Even though I knew my looks weren't appreciated by my schoolmates, it was another issue entirely to realize just how much they weren't appreciated by the world at large," she wrote. "The pit of self-disgust that I'd been digging since my cheerleading disaster was growing larger, darker, and much more depressing. It became the catalyst for a number of questionable future decisions as I grew increasingly incapable of accepting the beautiful identity trapped beneath my distorted expectations."

Jessamyn's first encounter with yoga happened around the same age Indra Devi had stumbled on it nearly a century earlier, though Jessamyn's initiation came with fewer daydreams and much more angst. Her jet-setting Aunt Tracy, "the epitome of glamour" for teenaged Jessamyn, was a longtime believer in breath work for relaxation, and in the early 2000s, she became devoted to what was then called Bikram Yoga.

Aunt Tracy invited Jessamyn to join her for a class. *You'll feel great after!* she gushed. Jessamyn reluctantly agreed—then immediately regretted it. "In a room full of advanced middle-aged practitioners, I was a fat teenage novice, and I stuck out like a sore thumb," she wrote. "About a third of the way into the class, I became convinced that my death by heat exhaustion was imminent. . . . I spent the rest of the class in a heap on my yoga mat, simultaneously trying not to cry and wanting to melt into the atmosphere."

Throughout college, Jessamyn would occasionally feel inspired to exercise, not as a path to empowerment but to lose weight. These fitness kicks were usually accompanied by dieting. It wasn't until her early twenties that she began to truly appreciate what her body could do for her.

The shift started when a bubbly and persuasive friend invited Jessamyn to try hot yoga again at a studio in Winston-Salem that was offering a deep discount for the month.

Her knee-jerk reaction: No way.

"I couldn't deny that I could use the exercise," she wrote. "I was actively looking for a way out of my emotional hole, [but] I didn't see how yoga could possibly help."

Eventually, though, her friend convinced her. Jessamyn borrowed her dad's old Pilates mat for her first class. She was terrified.

That initial class was as brutal as the one she'd taken with Aunt Tracy, physically and emotionally. "I remember feeling as though everyone's eyes were on me," she wrote. "And by 'everyone' I mean every single living and breathing human, from the person casually walking out of the studio to the bored studio receptionist to the person who chose to roll out her mat as far away from me as possible. (In my self-sabotaging mind, it was NEVER because they simply wanted to practice in a different part of the room.) Every single gaze felt like a judgment."

But she kept coming back. And little by little, through sweat and struggle, she began to gain some mastery over the postures. And most crucially, she began to trust her body. "That was a triumph all my own," she wrote, "a triumph I hadn't felt in years."

In the summer of 2012, just as she was making progress, she decided to follow her girlfriend to Durham, North Carolina.

(Jessamyn came out as a lesbian when she was seventeen and came out again as queer in her early twenties.) Without a job, she couldn't afford classes at the local yoga studios. She started practicing yoga at home and appreciated the freedom, but she craved guidance. It was the relatively early days of Instagram, and she was happy to discover its small yoga community. She began taking photos of her postures and posting them in hopes of soliciting feedback. That's when everything changed, she wrote. "I quickly found my place in this virtual community and with it, a sense of inclusion and encouragement I'd never felt in any live yoga class."

Without fearing other people's judgment, she found she could be fully present. "I couldn't have anticipated that I would fall madly in love with the simple pleasure" of home practice, she wrote. "Everything about the way I was practicing yoga felt unorthodox, and it was exciting. For the first time, I was free to wear whatever I wanted, hold poses as long as I wanted, and break a lot of rules. . . . I felt free to fall down, because there was no one there to see me when I hit the ground."

By posting photos of herself on Instagram, she also discovered that many people were shocked by her very existence as a fat yoga practitioner. "It was, 'Oh, my God. I didn't know fat people could do yoga,'" she told *Yoga Journal*. "And I was like, 'Why do you think that fat people can't do yoga? Fat people do all kinds of stuff *all the time*.'" She saw an opportunity to change the way fat bodies are perceived in yoga—and life.

She began studying everything she could about yoga, from its history to the evolution of its lineages to the ins and outs of human anatomy, and eventually she decided to become a certified yoga instructor. Along the way, she gained hundreds of thousands of followers, which led to her first book, *Every Body Yoga*. (It was published by Workman, the same house that published Richard Hittleman's yoga books in the sixties. The arc of history bends and stretches toward progress?)

Every Body Yoga is part memoir, part manifesto, part guide. It begins: "I wrote this book for every fat person, every old person, and every exceptionally short person. I wrote it for every person who has called themselves ugly and every person who can't accept their beauty. I wrote it for every person who is self-conscious about their body. I wrote it for every human being who struggles to find happiness on a daily basis, and for anyone who has ever felt overwhelmed by the mere act of being alive. I've been there. We all have."

The book sold nearly 60,000 copies, making it a certified hit.

In 2019 Jessamyn co-founded The Underbelly, a yoga subscription app through which she offers instruction. And through all of her platforms, she shares her guiding principles: Embrace life's messiness—the dark is as important as the light. Learn to be alone with your thoughts. Be yourself. And instead of asking yourself *How do I look?*, ask *How do I feel?*

She usually teaches in as little clothing as possible, often only her underwear. She's more comfortable that way, she says, and it helps to normalize what a normal body looks like. It also allows her to see her tattoos, which serve as notes to self. One arm displays the state motto of North Carolina, *Esse quam videri*, Latin for "To be rather than to seem." Another arm reads, "What I'm looking for is not out there, it is in me," a quote from Helen Keller, a personal hero with whom she shares a birthday.

As deeply grateful as she is for the status she's achieved—she currently has nearly half a million followers on Instagram—Jessamyn doesn't love thinking of herself as a guru or role model or even a teacher. In true yogi fashion, she sees herself as a perpetual student. She'd prefer the public see her as a best friend who loves yoga.

"I just practice trying to live my life," she told me. "I just try to show up in my life, and be okay when things don't go the way I thought they would, and be patient with myself and other people. . . . The real point of all this, the point of life, is to just be. . . . And if I'm teaching anybody, that's all I'm ever teaching."

But she does have a mission, and that is to make body-diverse classes accessible to anyone who wants them—and show the rest of the world why body diversity is so important in fitness.

Jessamyn's hundreds of thousands of fans suggest she's making inroads. As *The New York Times*'s Jenna Wortham wrote in 2017: "Although I am frequently the only woman of color in my real-world yoga and fitness classes, I can always turn to a screen and look at [Stanley] to remind myself that bodies like ours have a place in this realm."

During the pandemic, the at-home fitness giant Peloton also rose to become a powerful source of support for women of color who could afford its subscription-based services and equipment, thanks to its virtual community #BlackGirlMagic: The Peloton Edition. From early 2020 through mid-2021, the Peloton #BlackGirlMagic Facebook group exploded from 6,000 to 21,000 members, offering its members a place to connect over health- and fitness-related issues that hold particular relevance to them.

"I have never seen a space like this for Black women," Amira Rose Davis, a historian of Black women and sports, told me in an interview. "Black women have always been in physical spaces, both as participants and as people trying to exert control over them, but . . . [they've never really] had the opportunity to set the terms of those places." Until now.

Peloton #BlackGirlMagic's online discussions range from how to deal with hair and sweat (research has shown that hair management is a major deterrent to exercise for Black women) to the ins and outs of exercising with uterine fibroids, which are especially prevalent among Black women.

"One of the things that I like so much about the group," Davis added, "is that you get a sense of what other exercise spaces are missing."

Jessamyn Stanley's activism is part of a growing movement of radical body love. Over the past several years, she has been joined by scores of other fitness professionals—some of whom look like fit pros have looked for decades, some of whom don't—who are working to undo decades of cultural programming about how a woman's body "should" look. They are busting the myth that "inside every fat person there is a thin person waiting to burst out" and countering the argument that a woman can be happy only if she has a very specific kind of physique—a physique that is (surprise!) not biologically possible for most women. For those who find body *love* too much of a reach after a lifetime of shame, activists suggest women instead strive to cultivate simply "body neutrality." That is, acceptance—which is radical in its own right.

Since the early days of the fitness boom in the seventies and eighties, the cultural messaging around fitness—later adopted by American culture at large—has equated a person's outward appearance with their inner health. More than that, though, it has also equated the appearance of fitness with virtue, and any apparent lack of fitness, as measured by body fat, with moral failing. It has put the onus for health and fitness almost entirely on the individual.

This premise is flawed on just about every level, not the least of which is its lack of consideration for luck, genetics, structural inequalities, or environment, to say nothing of the decidedly unhealthy emotional anguish all genders experience trying to mold their body into a shape that is deemed "worthy."

But this hasn't stopped it from leading to widespread discrimination against women who veer from the cultural ideal. Research has shown time and again that "thin privilege" is real, and women who live in larger bodies are discriminated against in nearly every realm of society, from major issues—not getting hired for jobs—to minor ones—not fitting comfortably into an airplane seat.

Proponents of radical body love base their activism on more than simply a fight for a more compassionate and just society. It's also based on a growing body of scientific research revealing that Western culture's assumption that thinness equals health while fatness equals disease is . . . bogus.

The Health at Every Size movement is leading the charge to debunk this premise. Founded by Lindo Bacon—a researcher at University of California–Davis with a doctorate in physiology and master's degrees in exercise science and psychotherapy—the movement breaks it down like this: For decades, the medical community has treated fatness as a straightforward indicator of health, prescribing weight loss as a cure-all for whatever malady a fat person may be dealing with. But there is an overlooked X factor in the cause of disease among fat people, and that is the stress of living in a world in which some bodies are deemed "good and acceptable" and others "bad and unacceptable." Chronic stress is a risk factor for most diseases associated with obesity, including heart disease and diabetes—but in a society as sizeist as ours, stress is treated as secondary to fat itself.

The Health at Every Size movement doesn't claim everyone is at a healthy weight, nor deny that many diseases are more commonly found in heavier people. But its practitioners point out that research has not proven that weight *causes* disease—it simply shows association.

In their book *Body Respect: What Conventional Health Books Get Wrong, Leave Out, and Just Plain Fail to Understand about Weight*, Bacon and coauthor Lucy Aphramor argue that putting the onus for body size exclusively on the individual "reduces their ill health to poor 'choices' and blames them, all the while contributing to the stigma and judgmental thinking that fuels their oppression, worsens their health, and expands the health divide between the advantaged and disadvantaged."

In one study, researchers polled a group of more than 170,000 adults about their actual weight and "what they perceived as their ideal weight." They found that "the gap between those weights was a better indicator of mental and physical health" than their body mass index. "In other words," write Bacon and Aphramor, "body dissatisfaction, or feeling fat, has a stronger negative health effect than being fat."

Remember Dr. Kenneth Cooper, the father of aerobics? His renowned preventative medicine institute in Dallas, the Cooper Institute, has shown that the death rate for people who are "thin but unfit" is at least twice as high as for fatter counterparts who are fit. Bacon and Aphramor note: "Across every category of body composition, unfit individuals (and those with chronic disease) have a much higher death rate than those who are fit, regardless of what they weigh."

Despite loads of cultural messaging to the contrary, Cooper's research suggests that *fitness* is the key factor preventing disease—not weight.

Put simply, the Health at Every Size movement aims to help people "shift their focus away from changing their size to enhancing their self-care behaviors—so they let weight fall where it may naturally," write Bacon and Aphramor. By encouraging a more accurate understanding of health, fighting fat stigma, and promoting positive self-care, practitioners can address real health concerns, "giving both fat and thin people the support they deserve."

Body-acceptance activist Virgie Tovar puts it this way: "When you tell a woman, 'It doesn't matter what size you are—you could be any size and still deserve love and respect and dignity,' that is completely upending a very long history of misogyny."

It's a shift that is nothing short of revolutionary.

For all of these reasons, the new wave of fitness trailblazers see expanding access to exercise as a social justice issue, with the potential to help this country become not only healthier but also happier—not because of the weight people might lose, but because of the strength and well-being they might gain.

Cardio dance pioneer Sadie Kurzban, creator of the popular 305 Fitness, is helping to lead this charge. Since its launch in 2012, Sadie has grown 305 Fitness into a sensation among millennials and Gen Z exercisers, with studios in New York, Boston, and D.C., and licensed instructors across the country and around the world. Every high-energy class is meant to feel like a dance party—complete with live deejay or nonstop club mixes—and everyone's invited.

Growing up in Miami (the area code that inspired her business), Sadie was exposed to a host of toxic messages about women's bodies. There was the influence of the city itself, famous for its surgical enhancements and beach-driven focus on external appearances, which instilled in her unrealistic ideals about how a woman's body should look. ("I didn't know what normal boobs looked like until I got to college," she joked during our interview.)

But her home life had a more profound influence on her relationship with her body.

The daughter of a Cuban mother and a Jewish father, Sadie grew up the fourth of five siblings. Her mom and three older sisters all struggled with eating disorders. "I grew up with the Latin stereotype of a very sexually objectified woman who always thinks her man is going to leave, you know, and who only knows her worth as her body," Sadie told me when we spoke by phone. Still, her sisters hoped that Sadie, the baby, would be spared what they had suffered. They encouraged her to love her body as it was. "It was a lot of 'do as I say, not as I do.'"

But Sadie became fixated on monitoring her appearance, too. In fifth grade, she started counting calories, and by middle school, she was attempting to burn them off at the gym. "I would go after school, and I was super self-disciplined. I was following all the rules that the world had mapped out for me. You know, you go to the gym and look good and control your weight and all these things. There was nothing joyful about it."

But the big change happened when her gym started offering Zumba classes. She turned up her nose at the classes at first. "I just thought to myself, this isn't serious. It's not *exercise*—it's middle-aged women laughing," she said. "But the joy coming from that class was so real. And there was obviously a part of my soul that really wanted that. The teacher kept seeing me outside the room, and one day she just pulled me in by the forearm."

By seventeen, Sadie was teaching Zumba herself.

In her undergraduate years at Brown University, Sadie began offering the school's first-ever Zumba classes. "That community had given me so much joy and meaning and connection and safety and a lot of things I didn't realize I was so starved for," she said. "I felt like I had to do it." Over time, the class evolved. "I stopped doing the stop-and-start choreography. I hired a deejay, and it became more like a party." And then it became 305 Fitness.

From the start, she wanted 305 Fitness to be focused on joy, not weight loss or aesthetic transformation. Even if she hadn't been able to accept her own body yet, she hoped to do for other women what her sisters had attempted to do for her—*do as I say, not as I do.* "I started 305 as a way to teach us to talk to ourselves with kindness and encouragement," she told *Forbes* in 2019. "So many other fitness programs are about transforming yourself so that you can be accepted. At 305, we say: you don't need to change. You are perfect, just as you are."

When Sadie opened her first studio, in Manhattan's East Village, she made a point of hiring instructors from as many different back-grounds and life experiences as possible. "The face of 305 is Black, brown, white, larger-bodied, all genders, all orientations," she has said. Part of her sales pitch for her studios is that, because a deejay controls the music and every class has a slightly different playlist, the instructors are kept a little bit vulnerable—which she hopes helps her students fight the need to try to be perfect. "You know, you can show up and be confident and you don't have to get every single thing right in order to like yourself. We mess up in every single class. And it's part of the fun."

Beyond the classroom, Sadie has become a leader in the industry for proposing innovative ways the private sector can help level the playing field. While classes in her brick-and-mortar studios start at $32 per session ("The overhead of studios in New York City makes it actually just impossible to charge anything less," she told me), 305 Fitness also offers weekly "community classes" for half the cost. During the pandemic, the company launched a digital subscription service for $29 a month, with a sliding scale for clients who have faced hiring discrimination or are burdened with student loans or face other financial obstacles. And she gives clients the ability to pay it forward and anonymously cover other people's memberships.

Like Jazzercise in the early eighties, 305 Fitness also licenses in-structors who want to bring the classes to their own communities. "They go out, and they can teach in a park, they can teach online, but they can charge two dollars or five dollars. And that's what's re-ally cool—that these people are going to take it and make it their own." (*The Joy of Movement* author Kelly McGonigal is herself a certified 305 Fitness instructor. She teaches classes in and around Stanford University.)

Next up on Sadie's list of goals is adapting her classes to be inclu-sive of people with physical disabilities. "The way that I work out is obviously created with one kind of physical ability in mind," she says. "Something that's on our radar is creating a format that can work regardless of whatever your physical ability or physical disability might be."

Sadie says her larger mission is teaching people to "love themselves harder and express themselves louder, ultimately leading to empowerment." She adds: "Fitness is a path to that, but it's not the end result. As I think about how to build a better world for this next generation, we are only going to get there if we can 'arm the rebels.' But how do we get people to have the confidence to *be* that rebel and to think for themselves?"

With 305 Fitness, she hopes to help people feel more comfortable in their own skin. "When we feel embodied," she says, "we're more aware of what we need."

———————

The larger fitness industry is slowly catching on, and our cultural understanding of what a "fit body" looks like is evolving. Over the past few years, this body-inclusive mindset has even reshaped some major cultural institutions. Most women's magazines have stopped explicitly telling women how to lose inches and started featuring cover models in a range of sizes. And a growing number of major retailers, from J.Crew and Anthropologie to Old Navy and Target, showcase models whose size varies by more than just a digit or two.

Many fitness franchises have moved away from explicitly discussing weight loss and physical transformation linked to conventional standards of beauty, too. The co-founders of Physique 57, the popular barre franchise, told me that a decade ago, they openly discussed helping women get rid of their "muffin top" in their classes and videos—language that now makes them cringe. With some notable exceptions, fewer gyms openly promise a "beach body" or a "bikini body." (As body-positive activists say: Want a beach body? Take your body to the beach.) Workout wear brands have also gotten on board: Lululemon and Athleta and Outdoor Voices now feature models in a spectrum of sizes, as well as models with visible cellulite. Nike now displays mannequins with a variety of body types and abilities.

"There's been a buy-in, almost, from capitalism," says historian Elizabeth Matelski, the author of *Reducing Bodies*. "Big brands, big pillars of our social media mindset are kind of getting woke." This is not to say that corporate America's intentions are necessarily altruistic or noble. Many brands, of course, are simply capitalizing on woke culture, channeling the social mindset to sell things. Body-acceptance activist Virgie Tovar says she doesn't mind: "Either tactic, either motivation is fine, frankly. They can have their awakening later if they need to."

There are signs that our cultural appreciation for more moderate forms of movement is evolving, too. When the world shut down, the coronavirus pandemic shifted the way many of us think about our bodies and how we care for them. Confined to their home, some felt less pressure to maintain a perfectly toned physique. Others found that by shifting their workout from a public space to a private one, they felt emboldened to try new things—not unlike Jessamyn's experience when she bought her yoga practice home. And others have shared that exercise once felt like a chore but now feels like a luxury.

"It is so profound to me the gifts the pandemic has brought us," Jessamyn told me. "It was such a brutal, messy, nasty, violent, scary, hopelessly sad thing that happened. But at the same time, at the exact same moment, there are these incredible gifts, and one of them is that we actually value what it is to be in our bodies."

We may not see the measurable impact of this shift for some time, but for many, the simple act of stepping outside to breathe fresh air, of putting one foot in front of the other, feels like a victory.

Today, the first waves of women's fitness enthusiasts—the women who fueled the jogging and aerobics booms of the seventies and eighties and lived the history in these pages—are navigating their seventies, eighties, and nineties. It is through these women's experiences that we are—for the first time, really—beginning to get a sense of how the freedom and framework to sweat can shape the full arc of a woman's life when she is given the opportunity to move.

One of the great joys of researching this book was interviewing these women about the myriad ways exercise has expanded their perception of what aging can look like. Many grew up being told they had to stop moving when they hit adulthood—and watched their mothers stop moving—and don't take their continued forward motion for granted. Fitness has allowed them to hold on to perpetual youth. Not necessarily of the tight-skinned and slim-figured variety, but the kind that allows you to be an active participant in your own life.

Elaine LaLanne, the widow of Jack LaLanne, told me that as a young woman, she used to think, *I don't want to be old when I'm old*. Now, in her mid-nineties, she says, laughing, "I *still* don't want to be old when I'm old." Her exercise routine of walking and strength-training keeps her young of heart and body. "My mother used to say, 'I don't feel so old, but my feet don't want to go as fast,'" she told me. "But my feet go pretty fast!"

Joyce Hein, a retired seventy-two-year-old hospital CEO in Duluth, Minnesota, who still runs half-marathons, shared a similar sentiment of not wanting to be limited by age. "You know, I don't want to get into that stereotype of what a senior citizen does—that we just do our little social activities, our little church activities," she told me. "So many older women have a tendency to kind of close in and shrink the possibilities of what they can experience. Exercise helps you be more optimistic about aging." Joyce started running in her late fifties as a way to get in shape to climb Mount Kilimanjaro. She's since ascended the lower levels of Mount Everest in Tibet and completed the Tour du Mont Blanc trek in Europe. She has also run eight half-marathons and four marathons.

Most of the older women I spoke with initially started exercising to "get in shape"—code for losing weight and firming up their figures—but with time, they found movement to be both a tool for self-acceptance and a ticket to living a full life. As Jane Fonda wrote in *My Life So Far*, "Maybe in our Western culture you have to be a certain age for this to happen: to have lived long enough to love your hips for having enabled you to bear children, your shoulders to bear burdens, your legs to have carried you where you needed to go."

My mom, now seventy-two years old, continues to view exercise as essential to her well-being. After discovering aerobics and running in her thirties, she took up tennis and reveled in being active. Beginning in her fifties, however, her body began to rebel, forcing her to undergo multiple abdominal and pelvic surgeries.

"With each setback, I had to regain my strength and rebuild my stamina, but I never considered that I would become sedentary," she told me. "I wasn't ready to give up."

Six years ago my mom discovered a new physical passion—this time thanks to a Groupon for a local cardio dance studio. The first time she showed up to Dance It Off, she remembers, she saw "smiling women (my age!) moving, gyrating, jumping, and sweating to fantastic music." Several of these women have since become her dear friends. During the pandemic, she Zoomed into class three times a week. "I just know that moving my body feels great," she says. "It's a pretty simple equation."

Many women I interviewed talked about how proud they were to have set an example of physical strength and vigor for their daughters and granddaughters, an example they lacked in their own homes growing up. Some women told me about how their fitness habits inspired their daughters to become competitive athletes—a path that wasn't available to them as girls. Fitness titan Kathy Smith encouraged her daughter Kate Grace all the way to the 2016 Olympics in Rio, where she was the top American entrant in the 800-meter track event—the same event that, in 1928, was banned for creating "pitiful spectacles" out of women. "My mom had cheerleading available in high school," Kate Grace told *The New York Times*. "She is fitter than most of us, but of course she wasn't told [she could be an elite athlete]. But I was told it, and I believed it."

While writing this book, I have spent a lot of time thinking about my own motivations for exercise. I exercise to feel joyful and energized and strong. I exercise to manage anxiety. I exercise to feel proud. When I think about the times movement has made me happiest, these experiences have had very little to do with cosmetic transformation—training for and running a race, dancing, feeling my muscles strengthen in barre class.

And yet, so often after an exercise hiatus, the incentive that inspires me to get moving again is the promise of my jeans fitting a little looser and my arms becoming firmer. The promise of aesthetic transformation provides a convenient concrete goal—one that can be more fun, sexier, to think about than, say, working against a family history of heart disease or warding off back pain. Americans are deeply drawn in by makeover stories; what is the American dream if not a makeover story writ large? It can be hard to resist the lure of before and after photos.

Sometimes the promise of physical transformation can be the key that starts our engines, whizzing us off to more profound aspirations. But exercising to meet a cultural ideal of beauty can be a slippery slope. In our culture, which still sells women on the idea that there is always room for physical improvement, I try to remind myself that the deep, soul-nourishing kind of happiness I'm seeking doesn't come from molding my body to more closely resemble what our culture has deemed acceptable. It comes from feeling free.

Perhaps this is why one of my favorite discoveries while researching this book was learning that when humans move in sync with one another, we experience a kind of neurochemical alchemy that creates a feeling of collective joy. Researchers believe it grew out of our ancestors' need to cooperate for survival. Whenever a new group workout takes off, notes Kelly McGonigal—from aerobics to spinning to Tae Bo—it's because its creators have added one crucial ingredient: synchrony.

Researchers have discovered that when we move together, whether slowly during yoga or ecstatically in a dance class, these neurochemicals have the power to bond strangers and build trust. They increase pain tolerance. They also make us feel connected to something bigger—synchronous movement can create the physical sensation of boundaries dissolving.

"Somehow the brain is tricked into perceiving your body as just one part of a larger whole that it can sense in its entirety," writes McGonigal. Collective movement broadens our perception of personal space, creating "an expanded sense of belonging and an embodied knowing that you have the right to take up space in the world."

Perhaps this is why, in the first few strides of a road race, tears well in my eyes. Or why, the first time I joined my mom for her cardio dance class, I felt a similar swell of joy. In a world where we are so often out of sync with one another, for a fleeting moment, movement allows us to feel totally and completely connected to those around us. Imagine if everyone had regular access to this feeling?

Women's fitness may have caught on because of its promise to reduce us, but its true potential lies in helping every body become limitless.

Where Are They Now?

Bonnie Prudden never stopped evangelizing about "keeping fit," continuing to write, read, teach, and move for the full arc of her nearly one hundred years on earth. In 2007, she was one of the first recipients of a Lifetime Achievement Award from the President's Council on Physical Fitness, Sport, and Nutrition, the advisory group she helped create in 1956. "Every once in a while I have a conversation with God," she told a reporter in 1997. "I say I'm tired. This work is just too hard. Can I retire? The answer is always no." She eventually took a final bow in December 2011, when she died at age ninety-seven.

Lotte Berk continued teaching her barre-based fitness method into her late seventies. She also continued to take lovers. "Even as an octogenarian, her conker-brown hair shone with a rich, deep gloss," a *Guardian* reporter noted, "and with her dark eyes outlined in black, and bright with mischief, she could resemble a sexy gerbil." In her later years, Lotte liked to claim she had been married seven times, "twice on paper." She spent her final decade living in Hungerford, Berkshire, England, near her daughter, Esther Fairfax. In November 2003, she died at age ninety.

Esther Fairfax continued teaching the Lotte Berk technique out of her home studio in Hungerford until April 2021, when she finally decided to put away her whip. In the years since my feature story in The Cut was published, she has received a flurry of calls from journalists, documentarians, and filmmakers interested in exploring her and her mother's life stories. In June 2020, Esther published her fifth book, *How to Live and Die,* in which she "looks back with compassion and wisdom at her chaotic upbringing and strained relationship with her mother," and shares her "renewed purpose in training the next generation of teachers."

Lydia Bach's New York City barre studio, the Lotte Berk Method, shut its doors in 2005 after thirty-four years, amid intensifying competition from newer, plusher franchises—many of which were started by clients who had trained at the studio. "I've had to reinvent myself so many times," she told me in 2019. "I like challenges." Now in her early eighties, she stays active by sprinting up hills, stretching, and doing the Lotte Berk moves. She splits her time between the Hamptons and the Caribbean.

Kathrine Switzer has run more than three dozen marathons, and at seventy-four years old, she has no plans to retire from the sport. She also continues to be a tireless advocate for women runners. In 2015, she founded 261 Fearless, a global nonprofit whose name was inspired by the bib number she wore in her fateful Boston Marathon run. The group uses running as a vehicle to empower women "of all abilities to support, encourage, and inspire each other towards a positive sense of self and fearlessness." She and her husband, the writer and runner Dr. Roger Robinson, split their time between New York's Hudson Valley and Wellington, New Zealand.

Bobbi Gibb continued to defy society's unwritten rules for women when she forged a career as a lawyer and neuroscientist. She currently works as an artist—her primary medium is sculpture—and a medical researcher devoted to finding a cure for ALS. In 2016, with the fiftieth anniversary of her historic Boston Marathon run, Bobbi served as Grand Marshal of the race. More recently, a life-size statue in her likeness has been built and awaits installation along the marathon route. Bobbi splits her time between Massachusetts and Southern California.

Lisa Z. Lindahl served as CEO of Jogbra Inc. until its sale to Playtex in 1990. Since then, she has continued her work as an artist as well as a champion for women's health. Her advocacy work with the Epilepsy Foundation of America earned her a commendation from the U.S. Congress in 2000, and in 2001, she co-invented another novel undergarment: a compression bra for breast cancer survivors. In 2019, she published a book titled *Unleash the Girls: The Untold Story of the Invention of the Sports Bra and How It Changed the World (And Me)*. She lives in Charleston, South Carolina.

Hinda Miller remained a top executive in the sports bra business until 1997, then went on to serve as a Vermont state senator—an office she held from 2003 until 2012. She currently runs Deforest Concepts, a business consulting firm, and in her spare time, she works as an activist for women's health and entrepreneurship; she is also writing a memoir. She splits her time between Vermont and Florida, where she practices yoga and walks daily.

Polly Smith's decision to leave Jogbra for the Jim Henson Company was a fruitful one: She enjoyed a decades' long career as a costume designer for the Muppets, winning eight Emmy Awards for her work on *Sesame Street*. She lives in New York City.

Judi Sheppard Missett, now in her late seventies, still serves as CEO of Jazzercise, Inc., which remains the largest dance fitness company in the world, bringing in gross sales of more than $2 billion. Together with her daughter, Shanna Missett Nelson—who is president of the company—Judi continues to "manage and motivate" nearly 8,500 Jazzercise franchisees as well as choreograph and teach the program she invented. (In 2020, Judi's teen granddaughter also became a certified instructor.) In 2017, with the encouragement of then President Barack Obama and First Lady Michelle Obama, Judi launched a Jazzercise initiative called #GirlForce, which offers free classes to women between the ages of sixteen and twenty-one. She is the recipient of numerous lifetime achievement awards. She lives in San Diego with her husband, Jack Missett.

Gilda Marx oversaw her empire of Flexatards and workout fashion for twenty-two years. In 1996, she sold her company, then called Gilda Marx Industries, to Bestform. Since retiring, she has worked to support City of Hope, a National Cancer Institute, in its medical research. She lives in Beverly Hills with her husband, Bob Marx, where she still enjoys walking, lifting weights, and breaking a sweat in her home gym.

Jane Fonda, in her mid-eighties, is as passionate—and public—as she was when she first opened the Workout. A tireless advocate for environmental and social justice, she drew national attention in 2019 when she repeatedly got arrested while protesting in demand of more aggressive climate change policies in Washington. In 2020, she released a new book, *What Can I Do?: My Path from Climate Despair to Action*, donating all proceeds to Greenpeace. She stars in the Netflix comedy *Grace and Frankie* alongside longtime friend and collaborator Lily Tomlin, and in 2021, she received the Cecil B. DeMille lifetime achievement award at the Golden Globes. During the coronavirus pandemic, she even reprised her role as a fitness influencer, slipping into a leotard and leggings to demonstrate her classic workout moves on TikTok, to spread awareness about environmental causes. She lives in Los Angeles.

Leni Cazden is happily retired near Phoenix, Arizona. She and her daughter, Lauri Torgeson, exercise together almost every day.

Jeanne Ernst works as a personal trainer in Irvine, California, specializing in older adults. She and her former Jane Fonda Workout studio colleague Julie Lafond have been best friends for nearly forty years, and they recently launched an electric-bike-based fitness business together.

Doreen Rivera left Jane Fonda's Workout studio in the early eighties to teach her innovative stretching program around Los Angeles. She went on to star in the popular 1986 home video *Stretch for Life* and serve as a health editor for the original *Latina* magazine. She currently runs The Bodyful Mind, a holistic fitness class "designed to provide people with the opportunity to experience themselves from within."

Janice Darling closed her aerobics studio, the Sweat Shop, in 1986, when the injuries she had endured from her car accident eventually forced her to undergo a hip replacement and the business of running a studio became too taxing. She went on to become a middle school teacher and principal—but she never stopped moving. Over the past few decades, exercise has helped her navigate breast cancer, the loss of jobs, and the loss of her husband of forty-five years. "[Exercise] keeps me in touch with my sense of self and my sense of worth," she told me, offering "a feeling that I'm valuable. Even when you're alone, you're still valuable." Janice lives in Los Angeles.

Lisa Lyon stepped out of the public eye more than thirty years ago, partly due to drug addiction. By the mid-eighties she felt she had outgrown the bodybuilding arena, and she moved into performance art. She was later legally adopted by Dr. John Lilly, a controversial counterculture scientist most famous for his efforts to communicate with dolphins and his work with psychedelics; she and Lilly were also lovers. Lisa lives in Los Angeles.

Carla Dunlap continued to compete in bodybuilding into her forties. In the early nineties, she appeared on the ESPN fitness series *BodyShaping* and served as a spokesperson for Danskin alongside icons such as Nadia Comaneci and Kerri Strug. For the last thirty years, she has taught classical Pilates, and for the last decade, she has taught pole-dance-based fitness classes. "One of my philosophies is to live like water," she told me. "I will continue to flow and move around and be whatever that particular moment demands me to be." Now in her mid-sixties, she lives in Boca Raton, Florida.

Tamilee Webb, now in her early sixties, works as a private fitness coach in San Diego, specializing in baby boomers. She still produces workout videos, available online, and she delivers motivational speeches around the country. Her buns of steel continue to make her proud. "If I'm walking somewhere and it's at night, I'm not afraid," she told me. "I hold my posture up, I got my muscles, and I'm like— just try it. You'd be messing with the wrong woman."

Lilias Folan lives in Cincinnati, Ohio, where she enjoys spending time with her adult children and seven grandchildren. She continues to practice yoga as a way of life.

Indra Devi spread her yogic philosophy around the world until her death in April 2002, a month shy of her 103rd birthday. She spent her final few decades living in Argentina, where a single television appearance in the early eighties transformed her into a beloved national figure. In yoga circles, she is known as simply Mataji—Sanskrit for "respected mother."

Jessamyn Stanley remains an internationally sought-after voice in fitness and wellness. In addition to co-founding and starring in her yoga streaming app The Underbelly, she is cohost of the podcast *Dear Jessamyn*, co-founder of the North Carolina–based cannabis justice initiative We Go High, and a regular contributor to *Self* magazine. Her second book, a series of candid essays titled *Yoke: My Yoga of Self-Acceptance*, was published in June 2021. She lives in Durham, North Carolina.

Sadie Kurzban is as committed as ever to growing 305 Fitness into a force for social good. She splits her time between Miami and New York City.

Acknowledgments

Gloria Steinem wrote that the value of a movement is feeling its warmth and motion around us—that the warmth and motion are the means as well as the end. Working on this project has held a similar value for me. It has been a privilege to be surrounded by the warmth and motion of so many women while telling their stories.

I am so grateful to my editor, Michelle Howry, for her enthusiasm and vision, her wise edits, and for being a joy with which to work. I feel beyond fortunate to have found such a perfect partner in publishing this book. Huge thanks to Ashley Di Dio for her savvy editorial guidance; production editor Janice Barral; copy editor Nancy Inglis; cover designer Tal Goretsky; interior designer Elke Sigal; design director Tiffany Estriecher; Sally Kim, Ivan Held, and the rest of the wonderful team at Putnam, who brought this book to life more beautifully than I ever imagined.

My literary agent, Allison Hunter at Janklow & Nesbit Associates, took a chance on this project when it was just a kernel of an idea and waited patiently and graciously while I took eighteen months to write a proposal. Her excitement about the book in its earliest stages—and our bond over the subject—was the carrot that kept me researching and writing while caring for a newborn and navigating new motherhood. I am so grateful for her advocacy, guidance, and friendship.

This book was shaped with the help of a dream team of readers. Kara Cutruzzula, thank you for dropping everything to read chapters as they landed and sending back brilliant edits. You are extraordinary. Joyce Tang and Allison McNearney, I am so grateful for your sharp notes and encouragement. Erin Geiger Smith, thank you for being there for me every step of the way. Jessica Berger Gross, you were the very first person to suggest I write this book, when I shared my surprise that no one had told this version of the story. Thank you, my dear friend, for your support—always.

I am eternally grateful to my fact checker, Andy Young; discussing and honing the stories in this book with you was a gift. Freelance photo editor Erica Singleton provided invaluable support in preparing the photo insert.

This book would not exist without the work of academics and researchers who provided a scholarly framework for its narrative. I am deeply indebted to historians Shelly McKenzie, Elizabeth Matelski, and Jaime Schultz. The psychologist Kelly McGonigal's work provided a north star for me, continually reminding me why telling this story matters. Natalia Mehlman Petrzela, I am so lucky to call you a friend. You have inspired me, taught me, elevated me. Thank you for your support and graciousness these past many years as we have worked on our respective histories of fitness culture.

This book was informed by conversations with dozens of sources who shared their time, insights, contacts, and archives with me, many of whom are not mentioned by name in the book. Special thanks to Enid Whittaker, Ken Alan, Kathie Davis, Kathy Smith, Jan Todd, Kenneth and Millie Cooper, Elaine LaLanne, Letty Cottin Pogrebin, Steve Wennerstrom, Jo Fairfax, Jacki Sorensen, Christine Matter, Kenny Harvey, Gin Miller, Stephanie Coontz, Amira Rose Davis, Lauri Torgeson, Suzy Prudden, Michael Folan, Matthew Folan, Sandy Webster, Ellen Wessel, Elizabeth Goeke, Mariah Burton Nelson, Doreen Rivera, Susan Grace, Darcy Halsey Harris, Kit Fox,

Lisa Loraine Taylor, Al Valente, Bill Dobbins, Richard Ravalli, Melissa McNeese, Cal Pozo, Ernie Schultz, Dan Koeppel, Mark Hatzenbuehler, Paula Span, Gina Griffith and The Total Workout, Janet Rosenblum, Elyse Rudin, Jill Epstein, Tina Lynne, Lori Benjamin, Charna Nissenson, Mallory Sobel, Candy Sobel, and Claire Mintz. I am incredibly grateful to Jean Buchanan, Joyce Hein, Ronda Beaman, Dale Orman, Robin Dobler, Marianne Clark, Mary Edwards, Kate Silc, Patricia Burgess, Sheila Roley, Donna Botterbusch, and all of the women who spoke so candidly with me about intimate details of their lives.

I am so grateful to the authors of the biographies and autobiographies that helped to bring this story to life, including Esther Fairfax, Kathrine Switzer, Bobbi Gibb, Lisa Z. Lindahl, Judi Sheppard Missett, Jane Fonda, Michelle Goldberg, Jessamyn Stanley, and the late Patricia Bosworth. The work of journalists Haley Shapley, Daniel Kunitz, Jonathan Black, Gina Kolata, and Blair Sabol also informed this project.

Many thanks to The Cut for publishing my 2018 piece on the hidden origins of the barre workout, which served as a gateway to this book. Ruth Spencer's deft editing and packaging helped that piece reach a wide audience—and convinced me there was an audience for this book, too.

I am fortunate to count Jane Spencer and Geraldine Sealey as journalistic mentors and friends. Both of you have given me the encouragement I needed to tackle big projects time and again—including this one—and you have made me a far better journalist.

I am forever grateful for my mother-in-law, Lori Arkin, who not only served as a one-woman public relations machine for this project but also connected me with terrific sources in Los Angeles who lived the history in these pages. Biggest thanks to Bob Arkin and Aaron Arkin for their unwavering support and enthusiasm. My thanks to the Arkins wouldn't be complete without a special shout-out to

Oscar-nominated composer Eddie Arkin, my cousin by marriage, who just so happened to compose the music for two of Jane Fonda's workout videos and generously shared his experiences.

My deepest thanks to Shere-Kay Gordon, who provided essential childcare during many writing hours. Sher, we are incalculably grateful for everything you do for our family.

Dad, thank you for showing me the joy of movement and instilling in me a love of running. Your excitement, enthusiasm, and faith has propelled me not only across race finish lines but in every aspect of my life. Mom, thank you for passing along your love of language, reading drafts upon drafts of my writing, and offering such a phenomenal model for what it means to be a woman who moves. My sisters, Jackie and Juliet, thank you for inspiring me every day.

Finally, Daniel—thank you for being the best partner in writing, in weathering a pandemic, and in life. Thank you for the countless hours you watched our beautiful boy so I could write, for reading and editing chapter drafts the second I stopped typing, and for making my dreams come true. I love you.

Notes

This book weaves together firsthand reporting and both contemporary and archival research. Direct quotations that are not clearly identified in the text are listed in these notes.

Epigraph

vii **"A movement is only composed":** Gloria Steinem, *Moving Beyond Words: Essays on Age, Rage, Sex, Power, Money, Muscles: Breaking the Boundaries of Gender* (Open Road Media, 2012), 271, Kindle.

vii **"Exercise gives you endorphins":** *Legally Blonde*, Metro-Goldwyn-Mayer, 2001.

Introduction | Sweat

xiv **multibillion-dollar industry:** Ophelia Yeung and Katherine Johnston, Global Wellness Institute, "Move to Be Well: The Global Economy of Physical Activity," October 2019, https://globalwellnessinstitute.org/wp-content/uploads/2020/09/GWI_2019_Global-Economy-of-Physical-Activity_North-America_Download.pdf.

xiv **The workout was created:** Esther Fairfax (daughter of Lotte Berk), interviews with the author, October 12, 2017, and July 23, 2019; Esther Fairfax, *My Improper Mother and Me* (Central Books, 2010), Kindle.

xv **Barbra Streisand:** Julie Welch, "Lotte Berk: Stylish Dancer Who Became a Fitness Icon," *Guardian*, November 8, 2003, https://www.theguardian.com/news/2003/nov/08/guardianobituaries.artsobituaries.

xv **I wrote about:** Danielle Friedman, "The Secret Sexual History of the Barre Workout," The Cut, January 19, 2018, https://www.thecut.com/2018/01/barre-workout-sexual-history.html.

xvi **Before the coronavirus pandemic:** International Health, Racquet &
Sportsclub Association (IHRSA), *2021 Media Report: Health and Fitness
Consumer Data & Industry Trends Before and During the Covid-19
Pandemic,* February 2021, 4.

xvi **But it also led:** Lauren McAlister, "Here's How COVID-19 Has Changed
Fitness," Mindbody Business, summer 2020 (based on the results of a
Mindbody survey conducted in May 2020), https://www.mindbodyonline
.com/business/education/blog/heres-how-covid-19-has-changed-fitness.

xvi **doctors cautioned against:** Judy Mahle Lutter and Lynn Jaffee, *The Bodywise Woman* (Human Kinetics, 1996), 1–9.

xvi **sports bra wasn't invented:** Lisa Z. Lindahl, *Unleash the Girls: The Untold Story of the Invention of the Sports Bra and How It Changed the
World (And Me)* (EZL Enterprises, 2019).

xvi **slipped under the historical radar:** Two notable exceptions include
Daniel Kunitz, *Lift: Fitness Culture, from Naked Greeks and Acrobats
to Jazzercise and Ninja Warriors* (Harper Wave, 2016), "Chapter 9: From
Women's Work to the Women's Movement," 219–49, Kindle, and the
recent ongoing work of historian Natalia Mehlman Petrzela, PhD, as in
"The Fitness Craze That Changed the Way Women Exercise," *Atlantic,*
June 16, 2019, https://www.theatlantic.com/entertainment/archive/2019/06
/jazzercise-50-years-women-fitness-culture-judi-sheppard-missett
/591349/.

xvii **"For centuries women have been shackled":** Colette Dowling, *The
Frailty Myth: Redefining the Physical Potential of Women and Girls* (Random House Publishing Group, 2001), location 368, Kindle.

xviii **"Our bodies are the physical bases":** Boston Women's Health Book
Collective, *Our Bodies, Ourselves: A Book By and For Women* (Simon &
Schuster, 1971), 13.

xviii **"I come from a generation":** Gloria Steinem, *Moving Beyond Words:
Essays on Age, Rage, Sex, Power, Money, Muscles: Breaking the Boundaries of Gender* (Open Road Media, 2012), 93.

xviii **"For women to enjoy physical strength":** Gloria Steinem, *Revolution
from Within: A Book of Self-Esteem* (Open Road Media, 1993), 208,
Kindle.

xviii **"I've gradually come to believe":** Steinem, *Moving Beyond Words,* 97.

xix **Steinem herself began practicing:** Steinem, *Revolution from
Within,* 242.

Chapter 1 | Reduce

1 **"I've been around physical ed for years":** *Pat and Mike*, Metro-Goldwyn-Mayer, 1952.

1 **"America, manpower conscious":** Editorial, *Eugene Register-Guard*, "Girls, Too," July 7, 1962.

2 **after weekly appearances on NBC's *Home* show:** NBC Press Department, "NBC News from 'Home': Easier to Get Mothers in Top Physical Condition Than Their Daughters; So States Bonnie Prudden, Starting a Keep-Fit Series on 'Home,'" press release, May 31, 1957; courtesy of Enid Whittaker.

2 **Bob Hope, Jerry Lewis, Dear Abby's Abigail Van Buren:** NBC Press Department, "NBC News from 'Home': Bob Hope, Jerry Lewis, Beatrice Lillie, Paul Whiteman Among 'Home' Guests Week of June 24; Howard Whitman Will Present Report on Teenage Drinking and Suggest Ways to a Cure," press release, June 14, 1957; courtesy of Enid Whittaker.

2 **"We are raising a nation of children with muscles of custard":** NBC Press Department, "NBC News from 'Home': Easier to Get Mothers in Top Physical Condition."

2 **shot at her "fitness institute":** per Getty Images, https://www.gettyimages .com/detail/news-photo/august-5-1957-sports-illustrated-via-getty-images -cover-news-photo/.

2–3 **Once, when Bonnie was late to an appointment:** Enid Whittaker (manager of Bonnie Prudden's private archives), interview with the author, February 2020. This was a favorite story of Bonnie's.

3 ***Bonnie Prudden says:*** Bonnie Prudden, *Sports Illustrated*, 35–43, August 5, 1957.

4 **Politicians and pundits:** See, for example: John B. Kelly, "Are We Becoming a Nation of Weaklings?" *Reader's Digest*, July 1956, 26–28; John F. Kennedy, "The Soft American," *Sports Illustrated*, December 26, 1960, 14–17, https://vault.si.com/vault/1960/12/26/43278#&gid=ci0258c07fc00526ef &pid=43278—-017—-image.

4 **Gone were the days:** Shelly McKenzie, *Getting Physical: The Rise of Fitness Culture in America* (University Press of Kansas, 2013), 1, Kindle.

4 **The rise of the suburbs:** McKenzie, *Getting Physical*, 59–60.

4 **From 1950 to 1960, the country's suburban population:** McKenzie, *Getting Physical*, 59.

5 **three-quarters of families:** McKenzie, *Getting Physical*, 40.

5 **"Housework won't raise a bosom":** Dorothy Stull, "Be Happy, Go Healthy with Bonnie," *Sports Illustrated*, July 16, 1956, https://vault.si.com /vault/1956/07/16/be-happy-go-healthy-with-bonnie.

5 **Americans were eating more:** Amy Bentley, PhD (food historian and NYU professor), interview with the author, March 2020; Marisa Meltzer, *This Is Big: How the Founder of Weight Watchers Changed the World— and Me* (Little, Brown, 2020), 45, Kindle.

5 **Swanson introduced:** Kovie Biakolo, "A Brief History of the TV Dinner," *Smithsonian* magazine, November 2020, https://www.smithsonianmag .com/arts-culture/brief-history-tv-dinner-180976039/.

6 **The Time & Life Building that housed:** Michael MacCambridge, *The Franchise: A History of* Sports Illustrated *Magazine* (Hyperion, 1997), 95.

6 **By 1964:** Centers for Disease Control and Prevention, National Center for Chronic Disease Prevention and Health Promotion Office on Smoking and Health, "The Health Consequences of Smoking—50 Years of Progress: A Report of the Surgeon General," 2014, https://www.ncbi.nlm.nih.gov/books /NBK294310/.

6 **While the rise of vaccines and antibiotics:** McKenzie, *Getting Physical*, 85; Bentley, interview.

6 **Meanwhile, military generals:** McKenzie, *Getting Physical*, 43–44; see also "The Flabby American," American Broadcasting Company, May 30, 1961, https://www.paleycenter.org/collection/item/?q=john&p=387&item =T82:0692; Robert H. Boyle, "The Report That Shocked the President," *Sports Illustrated*, August 15, 1955, https://vault.si.com/vault/1955/08/15 /the-report-that-shocked-the-president; and many other contemporaneous reports on the subject.

7 **"The mere mention":** Boyle, "The Report That Shocked the President."

7 **"Whenever I get the urge to exercise":** There is some debate over the origin of this quote. While *Sports Illustrated* attributes it to Hutchins in the editor's letter of its July 16, 1956, issue, other sources attribute an earlier version to Mark Twain.

8 **During a 1956 radio interview:** Recording of this interview courtesy of Enid Whittaker, Bonnie Prudden archives.

8 **Davy Crockett:** Stull, "Be Happy, Go Healthy with Bonnie."

8 **She had been hyperactive as a kid:** The biographical section that follows (and the quotes therein) come from a detailed autobiographical presentation

Prudden created in 2006, which she casually titled the "Bonnie Book." A copy of the "Bonnie Book" was provided to me by Enid Whittaker.

10 **sprawling estate:** For more on the Hirschland family home: https://hirschland.com/2012/03/21/harrison-tarantara/.

10 **Bonnie's Roof:** For more about the climb: https://www.mountainproject.com/route/105801433/bonnies-roof.

14 **"We fell in love":** Bonnie Prudden private diary entry, courtesy of Enid Whittaker.

14 **hypokinetic disease:** K. Hirschhorn, B. P. Hirschland, H. Kraus, "Hypokinetic disease; role of inactivity in production of disease," *The New York State Journal of Medicine*, as cited in Boyle, "The Report That Shocked the President."

14 **"How Fit Are Our Children?":** Elizabeth Pope, "How Fit Are Our Children?" *Ladies' Home Journal*, March 1954, 69, 90–93.

15 **"Is your child a 'softie'?":** See, for example: "Is Your Child a 'Softie'?" *New York Post*, February 28, 1964.

15 **Bonnie had been teaching:** The biographical section that follows (and the direct quotes therein) come from the "Bonnie Book."

16 **Nearly a year after:** Boyle, "The Report That Shocked the President."

16 **On a balmy July 11, 1955:** Boyle, "The Report That Shocked the President"; Prudden, "Bonnie Book."

17 **"I don't see this country lasting":** Stull, "Be Happy, Go Healthy with Bonnie."

17 **The report was not without its critics:** Boyle, "The Report That Shocked the President."

17 **He gave the task:** Dorothy Stull, "Conference at Annapolis: First Blow for Fitness," *Sports Illustrated*, July 2, 1956, https://vault.si.com/vault/1956/07/02/conference-at-annapolis-first-blow-for-fitness.

18 **"Talk talk talk":** Stull, "Be Happy, Go Healthy with Bonnie."

19 **Once, when she was climbing:** Whittaker, interview. This was another of Bonnie's favorite stories to tell.

19 **"Under Bonnie's magic spell":** Stull, "Be Happy, Go Healthy with Bonnie."

20 **When it was illegal:** Stephanie Coontz, *A Strange Stirring: The Feminine Mystique and American Woman at the Dawn of the 1960s* (Basic Books, 2011), 11, Kindle.

20   **It hadn't always been this way:** Susan J. Douglas, *Where the Girls Are: Growing Up Female with the Mass Media* (Three Rivers Press, 1994), 45–46.

20   **"The war was over":** Douglas, *Where the Girls Are*, 47.

20   **By the end of the decade:** Daron Acemoglu, David Autor, and David Lyle, "Women, War, and Wages: The Effect of Female Labor Supply on the Wage Structure at Midcentury," *Journal of Political Economy* 112, no. 3 (2004): 497–551.

21   **Women were told:** Elizabeth Matelski, *Reducing Bodies: Mass Culture and the Female Figure in Postwar America* (Routledge, 2017), 31–32, Kindle.

21   **They married earlier:** Coontz, *A Strange Stirring*, 49–51.

21   **Besides, for generations, doctors had warned:** Judy Mahle Lutter and Lynn Jaffee, *The Bodywise Woman* (Human Kinetics, 1996), 1–9.

21   **Bonnie liked to say:** Whittaker, interview. Bonnie repeated this line in many of her lectures, according to Whittaker. "It always got a very good laugh and the point was made," she told me.

21   **It bears mentioning:** Jaime Schultz, *Qualifying Times: Points of Change in U.S. Women's Sports* (University of Illinois Press, 2014), location 3412–3524, Kindle.

22   **Another barrier to women:** Douglas, *Where the Girls Are*, 22; Matelski, *Reducing Bodies*, 115; Kathrine Switzer, *Marathon Woman: Running the Race to Revolutionize Women's Sports* (Da Capo Press, 2007), 15, Kindle.

22   **"A fat, passive nation":** Matelski, *Reducing Bodies*, 115.

22   **"It is difficult for modern American women":** Coontz, *A Strange Stirring*, 87.

23   **While the fitness industry:** Matelski, *Reducing Bodies*, 21, 121.

23   **Even Disney's animated heroines:** Marisa Meltzer, *This Is Big*, 44.

23   **America's Black communities:** Matelski, *Reducing Bodies*, 21, 174.

24   **In a 1953 Gallup poll:** Matelski, *Reducing Bodies*, 115.

24   **"Although reducing salons were not health clubs":** McKenzie, *Getting Physical*, 152–53.

25   ***Sports Illustrated*'s editors:** MacCambridge, *The Franchise*, 95–96.

26   **"Clothing is the most important thing at the start":** Petra Boncheff, "Bonnie Prudden: The First Lady of Fitness Fashion," *The Desert Leaf*, April 2008, 27.

26 **Bonnie was close friends:** Boncheff, "Bonnie Prudden," 49.

27 **journalist Gay Talese writes:** Gay Talese, "Women Prisoners Exhibit 'Fitness,'" *New York Times,* May 10, 1959, https://www.nytimes.com/1959 /05/10/archives/woman-prisoners-exhibit-fitness-25-at-the-westfield -farm-stage.html.

28 **Berney Geis had recently founded:** Brooke Hauser, *Enter Helen: The Invention of Helen Gurley Brown and the Rise of the Modern Single Woman* (HarperCollins, 2016), 17–18, Kindle.

28 **"publishing as a profession spoke":** Hauser, *Enter Helen,* 18.

28 **"trapped housewives and mothers":** Boncheff, "Bonnie Prudden," 26.

29 **Berney explained in a letter:** Berney Geis to Bonnie Prudden and Doro- thy Stull, October 10, 1960, courtesy of Enid Whittaker.

29 **Airlines pressured flight attendants:** Coontz, *A Strange Stirring,* 10.

29 **At Geis's encouragement:** Berney Geis to Bonnie Prudden and Dorothy Stull, September 29, 1960, courtesy of Enid Whittaker.

30 **The *Atlanta Journal*:** Letty Cottin, Bernard Geis Associates, "Reviewers are head over heels about two new Bernard Geis Associates Books!" news release, November 30, 1961. Courtesy of Enid Whittaker.

31 **"[Exercise] promotion efforts":** McKenzie, *Getting Physical,* 9.

31 **As far back as the early twentieth century:** Ava Purkiss, "'Beauty Se- crets: Fight Fat': Black Women's Aesthetics, Exercise, and Fat Stigma, 1900– 1930s," *Journal of Women's History* 29, no. 2 (summer 2017): 14–37.

32 **In 1962, an article in the trade magazine *Sponsor*:** Magazine staff, "TV's Great Bust-and-Chest Boom," *Sponsor,* October 8, 1962, 42–43, 54–56.

36 **women's bodies were projects:** See Joan Jacobs Brumberg, *The Body Project: An Intimate History of American Girls* (Random House, 1997).

Chapter 2 | Tuck

37 **"What *is* a sexy woman?":** Helen Gurley Brown, *Sex and the Single Girl* (Open Road Integrated Media, 2012), 128, Apple Books.

38 **As a design student in the 1950s:** Juliet Nicolson, "Mary Quant: Life, Love and Liberty," *Harper's Bazaar UK,* February 11, 2020, https://www .harpersbazaar.com/uk/fashion/shows-trends/a30873182/mary-quant -designer/; Jenny Lister, *Mary Quant* (Victoria & Albert Museum, illus- trated edition, 2019); V&A Museum, Kensington, London, Mary Quant

Exhibition, visited July 2019, https://www.vam.ac.uk/exhibitions/mary-quant.

38 **"Drinks for customers":** Nicolson, "Mary Quant: Life, Love and Liberty."

39–40 **"run, catch a bus, dance":** Nicolson, "Mary Quant: Life, Love and Liberty."

40 **"I didn't get fat":** Lisa Armstrong, "Mary Quant: 'You Have to Work at Staying Slim—But It's Worth It,'" *Telegraph*, February 17, 2012, http://fashion.telegraph.co.uk/news-features/TMG9087300/Mary-Quant-You-have-to-work-at-staying-slim-but-its-worth-it.html.

40 **"Until now it was fairly easy":** "Exercise," *Ladies' Home Journal*, November 1965, 94; Elizabeth Matelski, *Reducing Bodies: Mass Culture and the Female Figure in Postwar America* (Routledge, 2017), Kindle 47.

40 **"cotton and textiles":** Matelski, *Reducing Bodies*, 47.

41 **Born Lieselotte Heymansohn:** The biographical sections that follow are drawn from Esther Fairfax's 2010 memoir, *My Improper Mother and Me* (Central Books, 2010), Kindle, and Fairfax's 2017 and 2019 interviews with the author.

41 **"My life was filled with music":** Fairfax, *My Improper Mother and Me*, location 150.

41 **"I was tasting fame and loving it":** Fairfax, *My Improper Mother and Me*, 93.

41 **"Fear was like a silent fog that chilled the air":** Fairfax, *My Improper Mother and Me*, 183.

41 **In a conversation with her grandson in 1984:** Fairfax, *My Improper Mother and Me*, 190.

42 **"Hitler changed my life":** Fairfax, *My Improper Mother and Me*, 197.

42 **"She had such a natural instinct to flirt, to play the coquette":** Fairfax, *My Improper Mother and Me*, 1024.

43 **"Sex came into everything she did":** Fairfax, interview with the author, October 12, 2017.

43 **"Let's agree to forget about it":** Fairfax, *My Improper Mother and Me*, 425.

43 **"Cynthia was able to give her":** Fairfax, *My Improper Mother and Me*, 719.

43 **"I have got to do something":** Fairfax, *My Improper Mother and Me*, 912.

44 **suddenly found themselves rubbing elbows:** Fairfax, interview, July 23, 2019.

44 **he would play matchmaker:** Shawn Levy, "Oh, James . . . ," *The Guardian*, September 13, 2002, https://www.theguardian.com/film/2002/sep/13/artsfeatures.jamesbond.

45 **The world "needed somebody like Lotte":** Fairfax, interview, July 23, 2019.

45 **"It was all instinctual":** Fairfax, interview, July 23, 2019.

45 **"make something of it":** Fairfax, interview, July 23, 2019.

45 **a tucked-away road:** Description based on the author's visit to the studio's former address in July 2019.

45 **The studio was about a fifteen-minute drive:** Timed by the author during a visit in July 2019.

46 **Barbra Streisand:** Julie Welch, "Lotte Berk: Stylish Dancer Who Became a Fitness Icon," *Guardian*, November 8, 2003, https://www.theguardian.com/news/2003/nov/08/guardianobituaries.artsobituaries.

46 **"Go hang yourself":** Fairfax, *My Improper Mother and Me*, 912.

46 **"The classes gave women":** Fairfax, interview, July 23, 2019.

47 **"wicked tongue and sense of humor":** Fairfax, *My Improper Mother and Me*, 985.

47 **"Have you ever seen a flabby dancer?":** Fairfax, *My Improper Mother and Me*, 925.

47 **"muscles should be her corset.":** Fairfax, interview, July 23, 2019.

47 **"With Greta Garbo style":** Fairfax, *My Improper Mother and Me*, 979.

47 **For former Broadway and George Balanchine dancer Sandi Shapiro:** Sandi Shapiro (former Lotte Berk client), interview with the author, May 15, 2019.

48 **Sassoon had grown up in poverty:** Sassoon's biography in this section is drawn primarily from the documentary *Vidal Sassoon: The Movie*, Freestyle Releasing, 2010.

49 **"I work with the bones of the face":** Marisa Meltzer, *This Is Big: How the Founder of Weight Watchers Changed the World—and Me* (Little, Brown, 2020), 156, Kindle.

49 **"state of sex":** Fairfax, interview, October 12, 2017.

50 **"If you can't tuck, you can't fuck":** Fairfax, interview, October 12, 2017.

50 **"When photographed":** Fairfax, *My Improper Mother and Me*, 919.

50 **"I went to [her] for weekly torture sessions":** Prue Leith, *Relish: My Life on a Plate* (Quercus Publishing, 2012), 120.

50–51 **"Women had unlaced their corsets":** Fairfax, interview, July 23, 2019.

51 **"I was really physically strong":** Lydia Bach (owner of New York's Lotte Berk Method studio), interview with the author, October 15, 2017.

51 **"It changed my body":** Lydia Bach, interview with the author, August 20, 2019.

52 **who handed over the U.S. and Canadian rights:** Fairfax, *My Improper Mother and Me*, 2636.

52 **Later, according to Esther:** Fairfax, *My Improper Mother and Me*, 2636.

52 ***The New York Times* would showcase:** Angela Taylor, "From Shimmying to Standing on Your Head—Ways of Shaping Up," *New York Times*, March 24, 1972, https://www.nytimes.com/1972/03/24/archives/from-shimmying-to-standing-on-your-head-ways-of-shaping-up.html.

53 **she sent out hand-calligraphed invitations:** Bach, interview, August 20, 2019.

53 **Lydia told *The New York Observer*:** Rebecca Dana, "Battle of the Butts," *The New York Observer*, March 7, 2005, https://observer.com/2005/03/battle-of-the-butts/.

53 **"I felt that women should":** Bach, interview with the author, August 20, 2019.

53 **Tom's wife, Sheila, was a client:** Alexandra Wolfe, in conversation with the author, July 10, 2019.

53 **In that same *New York Times* article:** Taylor, "From Shimmying to Standing on Your Head—Ways of Shaping Up."

53 **In her 1973 exercise book:** Lydia Bach, *Awake! Aware! Alive! Exercises for a Vital Body* (Random House, January 1973), 87.

54 **The book's editor at Random House:** Nan Talese, interview with the author, May 20, 2021.

54 ***Cosmopolitan* gushed:** Lydia Bach, "Exercise Your Way to a Better Sex Life!" *Cosmopolitan*, April 1974, 36–38.

54 **"I loved the challenge":** Bach, interview, October 15, 2017.

54 **In a 1994 article for *Harper's Bazaar*:** Annemarie Iverson, "Body Diva: A Thoroughly Modern Lotte Berk Is Alive and Well with Abs of Steel at 81," *Harper's Bazaar*, February 1994, 50–51.

57 **Today, stand-alone barre studios number more than 850:** In May 2021, Pure Barre reported more than 500 franchise studios; The Bar Method reported 123 franchise studios; Barre3 reported more than 170 studios; and The Barre Code reported 60 franchise studios.

57 **Pure Barre's client base alone:** See https://www.purebarre.com/about.

57 **Journalist Samantha Matt wrote:** Samantha Matt, "I Took 500 Barre Classes—And It Totally Changed My Life," *Women's Health*, May 1, 2017, https://www.womenshealthmag.com/fitness/a19976401/i-took-500-barre-classes/.

59 **"I want that hour to myself":** Burr Leonard (creator of The Bar Method), interview with the author for The Cut, October 30, 2017.

Chapter 3 | Run

61 **"If you are losing faith":** Kathrine Switzer and Roger Robinson, *26.2 Marathon Stories* (Rodale Books, 2006), 106.

61 **At the dawn of the seventies:** Jane Leavy and Susan Okie, "The Runner: Phenomenon of the '70s," *Washington Post*, September 30, 1979, https://www.washingtonpost.com/archive/sports/1979/09/30/the-runner-phenomenon-of-the-70s/; David Lange, "Running & Jogging—Statistics & Facts," Statista, November 16, 2020, https://www.statista.com/topics/1743/running-and-jogging/; Jens Jakob Andersen, "The State of Running 2019," RunRepeat, March 2, 2021, https://runrepeat.com/state-of-running.

62 **Kathrine's mission began:** Kathrine Switzer biographical sections primarily drawn from Switzer's memoir, *Marathon Woman: Running the Race to Revolutionize Women's Sports* (Da Capo Press, 2007); *Boston: The Documentary*, Off the Fence, 2017, http://bostonmarathonfilm.com/; and the author's interview with Switzer, March 16, 2020.

62 **But Kathrine had run thirty-one miles:** Switzer, *Marathon Woman*, location 68, Kindle.

63 **"What are you trying to prove?":** Switzer, *Marathon Woman*, location 72, Kindle.

63 **They began playfully taunting him:** *Boston: The Documentary* (42:10).

65 **The 1928 Olympics in Amsterdam were partly to blame:** Rachel Swaby and Kit Fox, *Mighty Moe: The True Story of a Thirteen-Year-Old*

Women's Running Revolutionary (Farrar, Straus and Giroux, BYR, 2019), 31–36, Kindle; Amby Burfoot, *First Ladies of Running: 22 Inspiring Profiles of the Rebels, Rule Breakers, and Visionaries Who Changed the Sport Forever* (Rodale Books, 2016), location 100, Kindle; "In Amsterdam in 1928, Lina Radke Was the First Female Olympic 800M Champion, But . . . ," Olympic.org, November 3, 2019, https://www.olympic.org/news/in-amsterdam -in-1928-lina-radke-was-the-first-female-olympic-800m-champion-but.

66 **The *Chicago Tribune* called it:** As quoted in Roseanne Montillo, *Fire on the Track: Betty Robinson and the Triumph of the Early Olympic Women* (Crown, 2017), 83, Kindle.

66 **A reporter for *The New York Times*:** Arthur Daley, "In Praise of Greeks," *New York Times*, September 9, 1960, https://www.nytimes.com /1960/09/09/archives/in-praise-of-greeks.html.

66 **The Olympic decision would have ripple effects:** Swaby and Fox, *Mighty Moe*, 35.

66 **It didn't help that early twentieth-century educators:** Jaime Schultz, *Qualifying Times: Points of Change in U.S. Women's Sports* (University of Illinois Press, 2014), 1587–1594, Kindle.

67 **young women's track clubs were quietly springing up:** Swaby and Fox, *Mighty Moe*, 105–112.

67 **Flamin' Mamie's Bouffant Belles:** Gilbert Rogin, "Flamin' Mamie's Bouffant Belles," *Sports Illustrated*, April 20, 1964, 30–36, https://vault .si.com/vault/1964/04/20/flamin-mamies-bouffant-belles.

69 **Legend had it that a general:** Swaby and Fox, *Mighty Moe*, 124–26.

69 **quietly undertaking marathons on their own:** See, for example: Burfoot, *First Ladies of Running*, 22.

69–70 **"No girls ran in the Boston Marathon":** As quoted in Switzer, *Marathon Woman*, 117.

70 **he would "spank her":** "Lady with Desire to Run Crashed Marathon; Officials at Boston Shaken When Entry 261 Started Race," *New York Times*, April 23, 1967, https://www.nytimes.com/1967/04/23/archives/lady-with -desire-to-run-crashed-marathon-officials-at-boston-shaken.html.

70 **In 1966 Bobbi had crashed the marathon:** Bobbi Gibb biographical section primarily drawn from Gibb's memoir, *Wind in the Fire: The Personal Journey of the First Woman to Run the Boston Marathon* Institute for the Study of Natural Systems Press, 2016); other key sources include Burfoot, *First Ladies of Running* and *Boston: The Documentary*.

72 **"Hub Bride First Gal to Run Marathon":** See Amby Burfoot, "First Lady of Boston," *Runner's World*, April 6, 2016, https://www.runnersworld .com/races-places/a20791759/first-lady-of-boston/.

72 **"Boston was unprepared":** "A Game Girl in a Man's Game," *Sports Illustrated*, May 2, 1966, https://vault.si.com/vault/1966/05/02/a-game-girl -in-a-mans-game.

74 **Soon *The Tonight Show* with Johnny Carson:** Switzer, *Marathon Woman*, 118.

74 **Betty Friedan's *Good Housekeeping* headline:** Betty Friedan, "The Art of Living 2: I Say: 'Women Are People Too!'" *Good Housekeeping*, September 1960, 59–61, 161–162.

74 **There was the mega-bestselling 1968 book:** "The Art of Aerobics." *Time*, March 8, 1971, 60, http://content.time.com/time/subscriber/article /0,33009,904802-1,00.html.

77 **Pogrebin had written a bestselling:** Letty Cottin Pogrebin, *How to Make It in a Man's World* (Doubleday, 1970).

77 **women's movement leaders hoped to recruit Kathrine:** Switzer, interview, March 16, 2020.

78 **"And so, uh . . . you ladies are welcome at Boston":** Switzer, *Marathon Woman*, 168.

78 **"I let out a little cry":** Switzer, *Marathon Woman*, 217. For a visual, see https://www.gettyimages.com/detail/news-photo/jock-semple-b-a-a-boston -marathon-official-who-for-years-news-photo/515108138.

78 **"We were free to be athletes":** Switzer, *Marathon Woman*, 169.

79 **Fred Lebow:** Michael Janofsky, "Fred Lebow Is Dead at 62; Founded New York Marathon," *New York Times*, October 10, 1994, https://www.nytimes .com/1994/10/10/obituaries/fred-lebow-is-dead-at-62-founded-new-york -marathon.html.

80 **an exciting event he was planning:** Switzer, *Marathon Woman*, 174–77.

81 **the more running found critics, too:** Shelly McKenzie, *Getting Physical: The Rise of Fitness Culture in America* (University Press of Kansas, 2013), 116–18.

82 **The July 4, 1977, issue of *People*:** "Jogging for Joy," *People*, July 4, 1977, https://people.com/archive/cover-story-jogging-for-joy-vol-8-no-1/.

84 **"I ran quietly through the dawn mists":** Switzer, *Marathon Woman*, 330.

84   **The relay went smoothly until:** B. Drummond Ayres Jr., "A Relay for Women's Rights Runs Into Southern Chivalry," *New York Times*, November 4, 1977, https://www.nytimes.com/1977/11/04/archives/a-relay-for-womens -rights-runs-into-southern-chivalry-convention.html.

84   **In his book *Reaganland*:** Rick Perlstein, *Reaganland: America's Right Turn 1976–1980* (Simon & Schuster, 2020), 173, Kindle.

85   **Americans of color risked their safety:** See McKenzie, *Getting Physical*, 134–36; Natalia Mehlman Petrzela, "Jogging Has Always Excluded Black People," *New York Times*, May 12, 2020, https://www.nytimes.com /2020/05/12/opinion/running-jogging-race-ahmaud-arbery.html.

85   **America had a celebrated tradition:** Petrzela, "Jogging Has Always Excluded Black People."

85   **Jesse Owens was credited:** Quote from jacket copy of Jeremy Schaap, *Triumph: The Untold Story of Jesse Owens and Hitler's Olympics* (Houghton Mifflin, 2007).

86   **When the Black distance running pioneer:** See https://blackmara thoners.org/marilyn-bevans.

86   **"When some runners ran":** Anthony Reed, "The Pioneer: Marilyn Bevans," *Runner's World*, December 10, 2013, https://www.runnersworld.com /runners-stories/a20825589/the-pioneer-marilyn-bevans/.

86–87 **magazines intended for Black audiences:** See McKenzie, *Getting Physical*, 135; "Aerobics! Are the Perfect Exercises," *Essence*, June 1980, 84.

87   **Lisa Z. Lindahl started running:** Lisa Lindahl biographical section primarily drawn from Lindahl's memoir, *Unleash the Girls: The Untold Story of the Invention of the Sports Bra and How It Changed the World (And Me)* (EZL Enterprises, 2019); the author's interview with Lindahl, December 2, 2019; and Smithsonian Museum of National History archives, https:// sirismm.si.edu/EADpdfs/NMAH.AC.1315.pdf.

89   **"causing the pouch to stretch":** Lindahl, *Unleash the Girls*, 15.

89   **"Designers of bras":** Hinda Miller, interview with the author, May 20, 2021.

90   **Dr. Ernst van Aaken:** Switzer, *Marathon Woman*, 241.

91   **Judy Lutter's entry into running was not planned:** Judy Lutter biographical section drawn from the author's interview with Lutter on December 5, 2019; Pam Balcke, "Leading Ladies," *Runner's World*, October 1, 2001, https://www.runnersworld.com/advanced/a20818908/leading-ladies/; and Deborah Rissing Baurac, "Commitment to the Long Run," *Chicago Tribune*, May 16, 1993, https://www.newspapers.com/image/418164034/.

92 **tampon ads had shamelessly co-opted:** See https://flashbak.com/25
-vintage-feminine-hygiene-ads-that-offered-freedom-396964/.

95 **"bags and bags of Somewhere Cream Sachet":** Switzer, *Marathon Woman*, 316.

95 **"feminine touches":** Switzer, *Marathon Woman*, 318–19.

96 **When an official vote took place in 1980:** As cited in Jaime Schultz, "Going the Distance: The Road to 1984 Olympic Women's Marathon," in *The 1984 Los Angeles Olympic Games: Assessing the 30-Year Legacy*, ed. Matthew P. Llewellyn, John Gleaves, and Wayne Wilson (Routledge, 2015), 72–88.

96 **Reagan saw the Games:** Kenny Moore, "Hey, Russia, It's a Heck of a Party," *Sports Illustrated*, August 6, 1984, https://vault.si.com/vault/1984/08/06/hey-russia-its-a-heck-of-a-party.

96 **"ABC News had hired":** Switzer, *Marathon Woman*, 382–83.

Chapter 4 | Bounce

100 **would transform women's lives:** As described to the author in interviews; see also Natalia Mehlman Petrzela, "The Fitness Craze That Changed the Way Women Exercise," *Atlantic*, June 16, 2019, https://www.theatlantic.com/entertainment/archive/2019/06/jazzercise-50-years-women-fitness-culture-judi-sheppard-missett/591349/.

100 **By the early 1990s, nearly 30 million:** American Sports Data, "1993 Health Club Trend Report" (Hartsdale, NY, 1994), as cited in Beth S. Swanson, "A History of the Rise of Aerobic Dance in the United States Through 1980" (master's thesis, San Jose State University, 1996), 1, https://doi.org/10.31979/etd.8jv9-jyuk.

102 **1983 home workout video:** *Let's Jazzercise*, Universal Studios Home Entertainment, 1983; see also https://www.youtube.com/watch?v=uhR9f6KrK4k.

102 **a shyer Judi would emerge:** Judi Sheppard Missett biographical sections drawn from the author's interviews with Missett on January 24, 2018, and April 7, 2020, and on Missett's most recent book, *Building a Business with a Beat: Leadership Lessons from Jazzercise—An Empire Built on Passion, Purpose, and Heart* (McGraw-Hill, 2019); Swanson's "A History of the Rise of Aerobic Dance" was also a key source.

103–4 **jazz "emanates from the soul":** Missett, *Building a Business with a Beat*, 15, Kindle.

104   **"Gus's style was challenging":** Missett, *Building a Business with a Beat*, 15.

104   **"He said that what attracted him":** Missett, *Building a Business with a Beat*, 19.

104   **"By age 25, I was living my number one dream":** Missett, *Building a Business with a Beat*, 26.

105   **"They were there anyway":** Missett, *Building a Business with a Beat*, 29.

105   **"I hated seeing all the things I *couldn't* do":** Missett, *Building a Business with a Beat*, 30.

106   **"so long as it occurred":** Missett, *Building a Business with a Beat*, 32.

106   **"for me and for themselves":** Missett, *Building a Business with a Beat*, 32.

107   **"I believe five times as much muscle":** Quote from Dioclesian Lewis, found in Swanson, "A History of the Rise of Aerobic Dance," 36.

107   **"hardwired to hear music":** Kelly McGonigal, *The Joy of Movement: How Exercise Helps Us Find Happiness, Hope, Connection, and Courage* (Avery, 2019), 97, Kindle.

107   **The stronger the musical beat:** McGonigal, *The Joy of Movement*, 98.

108   **Catharine Beecher:** Swanson, "A History of the Rise of Aerobic Dance," 27–33.

109   **Made for just $3.5 million:** Simon Thompson, "'Saturday Night Fever' Director on Hollywood's $3.5 Million Gamble That Became Iconic," *Forbes*, May 3, 2017, https://www.forbes.com/sites/simonthompson/2017/05/03 /saturday-night-fever-director-on-hollywoods-3-5-million-gamble-that -became-iconic/.

109   **Disco deejays would come to influence:** Ken Alan (aerobic dance music producer who pioneered continuous track records for instructors; Body De- sign by Gilda studio manager), interview with the author, June 18, 2020.

110   **strikingly feminist article:** Rex Lardner, "Women Athletes: Tell Your Man to Watch Out—The Girls Are Catching Up . . . ," *Cosmopolitan*, April 1972, 206.

111   **One of the first Levi's for Gals print ads:** See https://www.levistrauss .com/2015/07/16/throwback-thursday-levis-for-gals/.

113   **"I was convinced that, unless I could be cloned":** Missett, *Building a Business with a Beat*, 59.

114   **"When was the last time you moved like a child?":** Judi Sheppard Missett with Donna Z. Meilach, *Jazzercise: Rhythmic Jazz Dance Exercise*,

A Fun Way to Fitness: America's Popular New Way to Fitness (Bantam Books, 1978), 1.

114 **"Give yourself room to grow":** Missett, *Jazzercise*, 13.

114 **"The fantasies you may have about being a dancer":** Missett, *Jazzercise*, 13.

115 **"Have you seen the kicks":** Missett, *Jazzercise*, 2.

116 **right behind Domino's Pizza:** See Michael Schroeder, "Looking for a Bigger Slice," *Lewiston Journal*, September 20, 1985, https://news.google .com/newspapers?id=EYlGAAAAIBAJ&sjid=kPIMAAAAIBAJ&pg =1507%2C2571118.

117 **"pilot fish at the nose end":** Daniel Kunitz, *Lift: Fitness Culture, from Naked Greeks and Acrobats to Jazzercise and Ninja Warriors* (Harper Wave, 2016), location 3451, Kindle.

117 **The Atlanta area had Arden Zinn:** A key source for this section of the chapter was Swanson's "A History of the Rise of Aerobic Dance."

118 **Jean Buchanan:** Jean Buchanan, interview with the author, February 10, 2020.

119 **"We experience *life* together":** Missett, *Building a Business with a Beat*, 168.

119 ***Essence* ran its first coverage:** "Exercise," *Essence*, January 1976, 46–47.

120 **the studio attracted a glittery clientele:** Gilda Marx, interviews with the author, December 4, 2019, and May 2021; Ken Alan, interview with the author, June 9, 2020; Gilda Marx, *Body by Gilda: Redesign Every Line* (G. P. Putnam's Sons, 1984). The latter discusses Marx's roster of celebrity clients throughout.

120 **Jules Léotard:** Nancy MacDonell, "Still Risqué, the Formfitting Bodysuit Rises Again," *Wall Street Journal*, November 27, 2019, https://www.wsj .com/articles/still-risque-the-formfitting-bodysuit-rises-again-11574857951; MacDonell (fashion historian), interview with the author, January 9, 2020.

121 **"I wanted to create":** Marx, *Body by Gilda*, 60.

121 **The story of how DuPont:** The section that follows on the birth of Lycra and DuPont is drawn from the work of anthropologist Kaori O'Connor, who gained rare access to the DuPont archives, and her 2011 book, *Lycra: How a Fiber Shaped America* (Routledge), Apple, as well as the author's interview with O'Connor on July 9, 2020.

121 **"During the explosives period":** O'Connor, *Lycra*, 157.

122   **"stable in price":** O'Connor, *Lycra*, 171.

122   **"In the period when Dupont":** O'Connor, *Lycra*, 197.

122   **Girdles were a "hallmark of respectability":** O'Connor, *Lycra*, 203.

122   **"There is no parallel in modern textiles":** O'Connor, *Lycra*, 199–201.

124   **"stretched and snapped back into place":** O'Connor, *Lycra*, 229.

124   **with the tagline "at last":** O'Connor, *Lycra*, 245–46.

124   **demand outran supply:** O'Connor, *Lycra*, 255.

124   **'Getting rid of the girdle':** O'Connor, *Lycra*, 267.

125   **"Its abandonment was political action":** O'Connor, *Lycra*, 279.

125   **"hugged the body":** O'Connor, *Lycra*, 311.

125   **"One day I looked at the back":** Marx, *Body by Gilda*, 59.

126   **Judi Sheppard Missett wore:** Missett, interview, April 7, 2020.

126   **"seemed to free the body":** O'Connor, *Lycra*, 316–17.

126   **Flexatards were a "harbinger":** O'Connor, *Lycra*, 319.

126   **"striking example of cultural blindness":** O'Connor, *Lycra*, 316.

127   **In 1984 alone:** O'Connor, *Lycra*, 322.

127   **"Lycra became the second skin":** O'Connor, *Lycra*, 314.

127   **rededication of the Statue of Liberty:** William E. Geist, "About New York; For the Grand Finale, Cast of Thousands," *New York Times*, July 7, 1986, https://www.nytimes.com/1986/07/07/nyregion/about-new-york-for-the-grand-finale-cast-of-thousands.html.

127   **"top woman entrepreneurs":** Missett, *Building a Business with a Beat*, 255.

128   **Jazzercise is now largely run:** Missett, *Building a Business with a Beat*, 154, 255.

128   **When we spoke at the beginning:** Missett, interview, April 7, 2020.

128   **"hundreds of thousands":** Marx, *Body by Gilda*, 25.

128   **Gilda collaborated with DuPont:** See company biography under Biography, http://gildamarx.net/.

129   **Gilda Marx just solved:** Gilda Marx (Gilda Marx Industries Inc.), *Vogue*, September 1989, 410.

129   **inspire Oprah Winfrey:** See "Oprah" video clip under Videos, http://gildamarx.net/.

Chapter 5 | Burn

131   **"Discipline is liberation":** This quote is widely attributed to choreographer Martha Graham, though the original source is unknown.

131   **"A good many dramatic":** *Barbarella*, Paramount Pictures, 1968.

131   **Carter's apparent weakness:** Shelly McKenzie, *Getting Physical: The Rise of Fitness Culture in America* (University Press of Kansas, 2013), 143–48.

132   **it was no coincidence:** McKenzie, *Getting Physical*, 143–48; see also Susan Jeffords, *Hard Bodies: Hollywood Masculinity in the Reagan Era* (Rutgers University Press, 1993).

132   **"muscles became a symbol":** McKenzie, *Getting Physical*, 145.

132   **1977 Gallup poll:** George Gallup, "Half of Americans Now Exercise Daily," Gallup poll news release, October 6, 1977; see also John Van Doorn, "An Intimidating New Class: The Physical Elite," *New York*, May 29, 1978, https://nymag.com/news/features/49241/.

133   **"I think of women's fitness history":** Ken Alan, interview with the author, June 18, 2020.

133   **Who was Jane Fonda in 1979:** Four essential sources for Jane Fonda biographical sections include Fonda's 1981 fitness book *Jane Fonda's Workout Book* (Simon & Schuster); Fonda's 2005 memoir, *My Life So Far* (Random House; Kindle edition); Patricia Bosworth's 2011 biography of Fonda, *Jane Fonda: The Private Life of a Public Woman* (Houghton Mifflin Harcourt; Kindle edition); and the 2018 HBO documentary *Jane Fonda in Five Acts*, https://www.hbo.com/documentaries/jane-fonda-in-five-acts.

133   *Redbook*'s **readers had recently:** Bosworth, *Jane Fonda*, 411.

133   **"All my life":** Fonda, *My Life So Far*, 737.

134   **"It was the start of countless":** Bosworth, *Jane Fonda*, 48.

134   **a "bore":** Bosworth, *Jane Fonda*, 43.

134   **"perfected an air":** Bosworth, *Jane Fonda*, 78–79.

135   **"Lady, if I gain":** Bosworth, *Jane Fonda*, 45–46.

135   **"an obsession with women being thin":** Fonda, *My Life So Far*, 119.

135 **"Starting my freshman year"**: Fonda, *My Life So Far*, 120; see also Jane Fonda, *Jane Fonda's Workout Book*, 13–14.

135 **"here's a way to *not* have our cake"**: Fonda, *Workout*, 14.

137 **The war had raged on:** National Archives, "Vietnam War U.S. Military Fatal Casualty Statistics," January 2018, https://www.archives.gov/research /military/vietnam-war/casualty-statistics; Ziad Obermeyer, Christopher J L Murray, and Emmanuela Gakidou, "Fifty Years of Violent War Deaths From Vietnam to Bosnia: Analysis of Data From the World Health Survey Programme," *BMJ* (April 2008), 336, https://doi.org/10.1136/bmj.a137.

138 **"What in the world"**: *Jane Fonda in Five Acts*, HBO Documentary Films, 2018, 0:30.

138 **"It's going to look like"**: Fonda, *My Life So Far*, 418.

138 **"That two-minute lapse"**: Fonda, *My Life So Far*, 418.

139 **"Putting his hand on my knee"**: Fonda, *My Life So Far*, 374.

139 **"I wanted a man in my life"**: Fonda, *My Life So Far*, 375.

140 **"Jane set out to make Tom"**: Bosworth, *Jane Fonda*, 397.

140 **move power "out of the hands"**: *Jane Fonda in Five Acts*, HBO Documentary Films, 2018, 1:23:12.

141 **"I was making one or more movies"**: Fonda, *My Life So Far*, 511.

141 **"keeping at least a tenuous connection"**: Fonda, *My Life So Far*, 512.

142 **"an enigmatic combination"**: Fonda, *My Life So Far*, 512.

142 **Leni dedicated the class:** Leni Cazden (former Gilda Marx instructor and original creator of the Workout), interviews with the author, July 11, 2020, and July 18, 2020.

143 **"strengthening and toning through the use"**: Fonda, *My Life So Far*, 512–13.

143 **"Up until then"**: Fonda, *My Life So Far*, 514.

143 **"I hated to miss even a day"**: Fonda, *My Life So Far*, 514.

143 **"You could open a studio, too"**: Bosworth, *Jane Fonda*, 437.

144 **"To be asked how I created my workout"**: Leni Cazden biographical sections drawn from interviews between Cazden and the author, July 11, 2020, and July 18, 2020, as well as Willa Paskin, "Jane Fonda's Workout, Part 1: Jane and Leni," October 13, 2020, *Decoder Ring*, produced by Willa Paskin and Benjamin Frisch, podcast, https://podcasts.apple.com/us/podcast/jane-fondas-workout-part-1-jane-and-leni/id1376577202?i=1000494513437.

146   **"The experience of teaching such a diverse group":** Fonda, *My Life So Far*, 515.

146   **"There will be a nuclear Armageddon":** Bosworth, *Jane Fonda*, 457.

147   **"It was like an avalanche":** Fonda, *My Life So Far*, 517.

147   **"Does it burn?":** Bosworth, *Jane Fonda*, 460.

147   **"No one, least of all me, ever imagined":** Fonda, *My Life So Far*, 515.

148   **An early promotional brochure:** Brochure courtesy of Janet Rosenblum, a Jane Fonda Workout client in the early eighties and a friend of the author.

149   **There was Jeanne Ernst:** Jeanne Ernst (Jane Fonda Workout studio manager and instructor), interview with the author, September 24, 2020.

149   **There was also Doreen Rivera:** Doreen Rivera (Jane Fonda Workout instructor, backup exerciser in Jane Fonda's first Workout video), interview with the author, October 20, 2020.

150   **Then there was Janice Darling:** Janice Darling's story drawn from her interview with the author, April 20, 2021, as well as Fonda, *Jane Fonda's Workout Book* and Paula S. White, "Tough Stuff!," *Essence*, September 1982.

150   **"Being in good shape is not just looking good":** Fonda, *Jane Fonda's Workout Book*, 48.

151   **critics pointed out:** See Bettijane Levine, "Jane Fonda: Working It Out," *Los Angeles Times*, September 14, 1979.

151   **The former Jane Fonda Workout studio regulars:** Special thanks to Jeanne Ernst, Julie Lafond, Doreen Rivera, Janice Darling, Ronda Beaman, Janet Rosenblum, Mallory Sobel, Gerry Puhara, Elyse Rudin, and Robert Aruj, for sharing their memories for this section.

151   **When *Los Angeles Times* writer Pearl Rowe:** Pearl Rowe, "Beauty or the Feast," *Los Angeles Times*, January 27, 1980.

152   **"We were there to do fitness":** Jeanne Ernst, interview, September 24, 2020.

152   **"got along wonderfully":** John Blades, "A Writer's Best Friend," *Chicago Tribune*, October 26, 1990.

152   **While working on the book:** Nan Talese, interview with the author, May 20, 2021.

152   **"Like a great many women":** Fonda, *Jane Fonda's Workout Book*, 9.

153   **she decided to write the book:** Fonda, *Jane Fonda's Workout Book*, 10.

153 **"break the 'weaker sex' mold":** Fonda, *Jane Fonda's Workout Book*, 45.

153 **"Please remember that your goal":** Fonda, *Jane Fonda's Workout Book*, 64.

153 **"There are no short cuts":** Fonda, *Jane Fonda's Workout Book*, 55.

153 **"frantically busy schedule":** Fonda, *Jane Fonda's Workout Book*, 56.

154 **"No audience could watch Jane":** Richard Corliss, "Sexes: On Golden Fonda," *Time*, August 30, 1982, http://content.time.com/time/subscriber /article/0,33009,921279,00.html.

154 **"threw Jane a champagne party":** Bosworth, *Jane Fonda*, 478.

154 **The device had made its American debut:** Priya Ganapati, "June 4, 1977: VHS Comes to America," *Wired*, June 4, 2010, https://www.wired .com/2010/06/0604vhs-ces/.

154 *Star Wars*: Jake Rossen, "How Jane Fonda Conquered the World," *Mental Floss*, June 19, 2015, https://www.mentalfloss.com/article/65314/how-jane -fondas-workout-conquered-world.

155 **Stuart Karl had a vision:** Essential sources for Karl section include Fonda, *My Life So Far*; Richard W. Stevenson, "Troubled Entrepreneur: Stuart Karl; From Fonda and Hart to Flops and Hot Water," *New York Times*, February 7, 1988, https://www.nytimes.com/1988/02/07/business /troubled-entrepreneur-stuart-karl-from-fonda-and-hart-to-flops-and-hot -water.html; "Jane Fonda's Video Victory," *Billboard*, August 31, 1985; and Rossen, "Jane Fonda," *Mental Floss*.

156 **"She'd never done video":** Michele Willens, "Jane Fonda: A More Personal View," *Billboard*, August 31, 1985.

157 **"we could sense the groundswell":** "Jane Fonda's Video Victory," *Billboard*.

158 **widespread injuries:** Kathie Davis (co-founder of IDEA Health & Fitness), interview with the author, September 14, 2020.

158 **She also reached out to Dr. Ken Cooper:** Kenneth Cooper (author, *Aerobics*), interview with the author, July 13, 2020.

159 **"You do the best with what you've got":** Jeanne Ernst, interview, September 24, 2020.

159 **When they did wear sneakers:** Key sources in Reebok section include Nicholas Smith, *Kicks: The Great American Story of Sneakers* (Crown, 2018); and J. B. Strasser and Laurie Becklund, *Swoosh: The Unauthorized Story of Nike, and the Men Who Played There* (HarperCollins, 1992).

161 **"doing Jane" in Cairo, Egypt:** Kate Silc, interview with the author, February 4, 2020.

161 **"When your voice and image":** Fonda, *My Life So Far*, 523.

161 **"What about me as an actor?":** Fonda, *My Life So Far*, 523.

161 **Debbie Rosas:** Beth S. Swanson, "A History of the Rise of Aerobic Dance in the United States Through 1980" (master's thesis, San Jose State University, 1996), 106–107, https://doi.org/10.31979/etd.8jv9-jyuk.

162 **"By the 1980s, advertising agencies":** Susan J. Douglas, *Where the Girls Are: Growing Up Female with the Mass Media* (Three Rivers Press, 1994), 245.

162 **"In stark contrast":** Douglas, *Where the Girls Are*, 245.

163 **"She drove her own car":** Julie Lafond (former Workout CEO), interview with the author, September 24, 2020.

163 **"When it was time to have lunch":** Gerry Puhara (Jane Fonda workout video costume director, mid-1980s), interview with the author, October 5, 2020.

163 **series of multimillion-dollar lawsuits:** UPI, "Jane Fonda and Her Spa Charged with Sex Bias," *New York Times*, March 31, 1983, https://www.nytimes.com/1983/03/31/us/around-the-nation-jane-fonda-and-her-spa-charged-with-sex-bias.html; "Jane Fonda Sued by Former Workout Instructor," Associated Press, October 14, 1987, https://apnews.com/article/fadb9d1fbe1fbe950424fe477af7ff40.

164 **"ripping her off":** Bosworth, *Jane Fonda*, 480.

164 **"Jane actually helped me":** Gilda Marx, interview with the author, December 4, 2019.

164 **"There was something about":** *Jane Fonda in Five Acts*, 1:26:20.

164 **"I had stopped bingeing and purging":** Fonda, *My Life So Far*, 738.

164 **"Hayden's campaign had been":** Bosworth, *Jane Fonda*, 476.

165 **"exercise in vanity":** Fonda, *My Life So Far*, 526.

165 **"Tom hated, loathed, despised":** Bosworth, *Jane Fonda*, 483.

165 **"Tom's the intelligent one":** Bosworth, *Jane Fonda*, 482.

165 **"It was purely a business decision":** Julie Lafond, interview, September 24, 2020.

165 **"I felt we had more than fulfilled":** Fonda, *My Life So Far*, 525.

165   **"An era in exercise has ended":** Alan Citron, "No Sweat: Jane Fonda Closes Her Beverly Hills Aerobics Studio," *Los Angeles Times*, April 3, 1991, https://www.latimes.com/archives/la-xpm-1991-04-03-fi-1696-story.html.

166   **"She found out about real people":** Julie Lafond, interview, September 24, 2020.

166   **"No one had prepared me":** Fonda, *My Life So Far*, 717.

167   **"Leni had been robbed":** Fonda, *My Life So Far*, 516.

167   **Jane also compensated her financially:** Paskin, "Jane Fonda's Workout," 45:00.

168   **"It's nuts that I should end up happy":** Paskin, "Jane Fonda's Workout, Part 1," 53:00.

168   **"Perfect is for God":** Fonda, *My Life So Far*, 120.

168   **"I had no idea what to expect":** Fonda, *My Life So Far*, 730.

168   **"I'm glad that I look good":** *Jane Fonda in Five Acts*, 1:58:48.

169   **Debbie also launched:** Jack McCallum, "Everybody's Doin' It," *Sports Illustrated*, December 3, 1984, https://vault.si.com/vault/1984/12/03/everybodys-doin-it.

170   **Also in 1983:** Charles L. Sanders, "Jayne and Leon: Did Success Break Up Their 10-Year Marriage?" *Ebony*, January 1982, 116–22; Laura B. Randolph, "Jayne Kennedy: Portrait of a Woman Who Lost Her Husband and Found Herself," *Ebony*, July 1983, 107–12; Doug Mead, "Twelve Women Who Pioneered the Era of Female Sports Broadcasters," Bleacher Report, August 21, 2010, https://bleacherreport.com/articles/440556-twelve-women-who-pioneered-the-era-of-female-sports-broadcasters.

170   **"I want every one of you out there":** *Love Your Body: Jayne Kennedy's Total Health Care Concept*, RCA Columbia Home Video, 1983; see also https://www.youtube.com/watch?v=Y1AncOS59-o.

171   **nearly *five hundred* workout videos:** Olivia Babler, "Survival of the Fittest: Home Exercise, Moving Image Technology, and Audiovisual Preservation" (master's thesis, Ryerson University, 2017), 45, https://digital.library.ryerson.ca/islandora/object/RULA%3A7140.

Chapter 6 | Lift

173   **"I have a head for business":** *Working Girl*, Twentieth Century Fox, 1988.

173   **When Lisa Lyon slipped into a bikini:** Essential sources for the chapter opener include Ann Salisbury, "New Breed of Body Builders Offers

Alternate Femininity," *The Daily Advertiser* (Lafayette, Louisiana), August 27, 1979; Eve Babitz, "The Girl from Gold's Gym," *Esquire*, October 1, 1979, https://classic.esquire.com/article/1979/10/1/the-girl-from-golds-gym; UPI, "Lisa May Be Little But Isn't Muggable," *The Daily Herald* (Provo, Utah), October 28, 1979; UPI, "Women's Bodybuilding to Become a National Sport?" *Town Talk* (Alexandria, Louisiana), April 5, 1980; Tony Kornheiser, "Lady in Weighting," *Washington Post*, May 27, 1981, https://www.washingtonpost.com/archive/lifestyle/1981/05/27/lady-in-weighting/9b30198a-cc20-492d-9f80-2f366512eb0d/; Lisa Lyon and Douglas Kent Hall, *Lisa Lyon's Body Magic: A Total Program of Body Conditioning by the First World Women's Bodybuilding Champion* (Bantam, 1981), 170–71; Richard Ravalli, "Body Magic: The Feminist Workings of Lisa Lyon, Female Bodybuilding's First Celebrity." Physical Cultures of the Body Conference, University of Texas, Austin, January 15, 2021; and Steve Wennerstrom (women's bodybuilding historian), interview with the author, April 7, 2021.

174 **"Except for her sculptured biceps":** Babitz, "Girl from Gold's Gym."

174 **"I look at my body":** UPI, "Women's Bodybuilding to Become a National Sport?"

175 **"Just to give you an idea":** Gloria Steinem, *Moving Beyond Words: Essays on Age, Rage, Sex, Power, Money, Muscles: Breaking the Boundaries of Gender* (Open Road Media, 2012), 97.

175 **"orthodontist to the stars":** John Lombardi, "Little Miss Dangerous," *Spy*, October 1991.

175 **she was frail and shy:** Lyon and Hall, *Lisa Lyon's Body Magic*, 1; Babitz, "Girl from Gold's Gym."

175 **"esoteric":** UPI, "Lisa May Be Little."

175 **One night on the campus:** Robert Mapplethorpe, text by Bruce Chatwin, *Lady, Lisa Lyon* (Viking, 1983), 13.

176 **"Here was something I could create":** UPI, "Lisa May Be Little."

176 **convinced the management:** Lyon and Hall, *Lisa Lyon's Body Magic*, 2.

176 **"A lot of the men bodybuilders":** Kornheiser, "Lady in Weighting."

177 **he worried "if he said the wrong thing":** Lyon and Hall, *Lisa Lyon's Body Magic*, 1.

177 **"Lisa had transformed herself":** Lyon and Hall, *Lisa Lyon's Body Magic*, 1–2.

177 **"Look at the latissimus!":** Lyon and Hall, *Lisa Lyon's Body Magic*, 5.

177 **"When I met Arnold Schwarzenegger":** Babitz, "Girl from Gold's Gym."

177 **had a job reading books and scripts:** Babitz, "Girl from Gold's Gym."

177 **courted by actor Jack Nicholson:** Lombardi, "Little Miss Dangerous."

177 **The International Federation of Bodybuilding asked Lisa:** Brenda Ingersoll, "Women Muscle Into New Sport," *Minneapolis Star*, December 11, 1979; UPI, "Women's Bodybuilding to Become a National Sport?"

177 **"In every era, the definition":** "She Gives Feminine Fitness a Lift," *Chicago Tribune*, October 26, 1979.

178 **In 1980, *Sports Illustrated*'s Dan Levin wrote:** Dan Levin, "Here She Is, Miss, Well, What?" *Sports Illustrated*, March 17, 1980, https://vault.si.com/vault/1980/03/17/here-she-is-miss-well-what.

178 **"There are still millions":** Kornheiser, "Lady in Weighting."

179 **"change her name to avoid":** Kornheiser, "Lady in Weighting."

179 **"Though standards of beauty for women":** Charles Gaines and George Butler, *Pumping Iron II: The Unprecedented Woman* (Simon & Schuster, 1984), 19.

179 **if you *did* want to spot a strong woman:** Haley Shapley, *Strong Like Her: A Celebration of Rule Breakers, History Makers, and Unstoppable Athletes* (Gallery Books, 2020), 53–61.

179 **Incidentally, the circus fostered:** Shapley, *Strong Like Her*, 53–61.

180 **a dazzling blonde named Abbye "Pudgy" Stockton:** Key sources for Pudgy Stockton biographical section include Jan Todd, PhD, "The Legacy of Pudgy Stockton," *Iron Game History* 2, no. 1 (October 1992): 5–7; Shapley, *Strong Like Her*, 67–75; Marla Matzer Rose, *Muscle Beach: Where the Best Bodies in the World Started a Fitness Revolution* (LA Weekly Books for St. Martin's Press, 2001); and Elizabeth McCracken, "The Belle of the Barbell," *New York Times*, December 31, 2006, https://www.nytimes.com/2006/12/31/magazine/31stockton.t.html.

181 **"women's bodybuilding, 1980 style":** Levin, "Here She Is."

181 **As early as 1971, *Our Bodies, Ourselves*:** Boston Women's Health Book Collective, *Our Bodies, Ourselves: A Book By and For Women* (Simon & Schuster, 1971), 117.

181 **"Weightlifting gives you confidence in yourself":** Carol Krucoff, "Supper Fitness: Bar Belles," *Washington Post*, July 14, 1980, https://www.washingtonpost.com/archive/lifestyle/1980/07/14/supper-fitness-bar-belles/.

181 **"Men have been doing this for a long time":** Brenda Ingersoll, "'Bar Belle' Set Here Small, But Participants Call It 'Uplifting,'" *Minneapolis Star*, December 11, 1979.

182 **"women's libber":** See, for example: Gail Mezey, "How to Treat a Lady Lyon: Respectfully," *St. Louis Post-Dispatch*, August 29, 1979.

182 **NBC signed her as an on-camera:** Lombardi, "Little Miss Dangerous."

182 **"The 1980s is the era of total womanhood":** UPI, "Women's Body Building to Become a National Sport?"

182 **"As far as long-term goals":** Gail Mezey, "How to Treat a Lady."

182 **She bought tubes of liquid graphite:** Mapplethorpe, *Lady*, 12.

183 **"The fact is, I didn't need another picture":** Kornheiser, "Lady in Weighting."

183 **Gloria Steinem later noted:** Gloria Steinem, *Moving Beyond Words: Essays on Age, Rage, Sex, Power, Money, Muscles: Breaking the Boundaries of Gender* (Open Road Media, 2012), 101.

183 **There was Lisa as "bride, broad":** Mapplethorpe, *Lady*, 14.

183 **workout wear line at Kmart:** See "All the News That's Fit," *Seventeen*, August 1990, 132; advertisement: Kmart Corporation, *Redbook*, June 1993, 18–19.

184 **Or by the women's magazines:** See, for example, "Muscles Go to the Movies," *Vogue*, June 1984, 304, and Susan Ryan Jordan, "Overcoming My Mastectomy with Bodybuilding," *Cosmopolitan*, November 1985, 224, 226.

184 **emerging scientific studies:** See "Spanning the Years," *IDEA Fitness Journal*, July–August 2017, 20, https://www.ideafit.com/wp-content/uploads/files/IDEA-35year-timeline-01.pdf.16.9.

184 ***Shape*, the first magazine:** Special thanks to Jan Todd (co-director of the H. J. Lutcher Stark Center for Physical Culture and Sports at the University of Texas at Austin) for contextualizing the birth of *Shape* in an interview with the author, January 24, 2021.

184 **"Body building makes you feel strong":** "Getting Strong: How to Shed Habits That Weigh You Down," *Essence*, October 1985, 52–56.

184 **When we spoke for this book:** Carla Dunlap, interview with the author, May 1, 2021.

185 **Henry McGhee:** See Jan Todd and Désirée Harguess, "Doris Barrilleaux and the Beginnings of Modern Women's Bodybuilding," *Iron Game History* 11, no. 4 (January 2012): 11–12; Levin, "Here She Is"; Conor Heffernan,

"Weight Training Women Stay in Shape Without Getting Muscle-Bound," *Jet*, September 1977.

185   *Time* **magazine ran a cover story:** Richard Corliss, "Coming on Strong," *Time*, August 30, 1982.

186   **"you're not condemned":** Kornheiser, "Lady in Weighting."

186   **"I started this sport":** Gaines and Butler, *Pumping Iron II*, 46.

186   **"Tough Women":** Kay Larson, "Tough Women," *Vogue*, October 1983, 222.

187   **executives told contest organizers:** Gaines and Butler, *Pumping Iron II*, 46.

187   **"third place":** See Ray Oldenburg, *The Great Good Place: Cafes, Coffee Shops, Bookstores, Bars, Hair Salons, and Other Hangouts at the Heart of a Community*, 3rd ed. (Marlowe & Company, 1999).

187   **"with sweating their form":** Blair Sabol, *The Body of America: An Insider's Journey Through the Bumps & Pumps, Groans & Moans, Pecs & Wrecks, Sweat & Sex of the Fitness Explosion* (Arbor House, 1986), 127.

188   **"Health clubs aren't just clubs":** Sabol, *Body of America*, 128.

188   **"At the bars, you look like you're":** Aaron Latham, "Looking for Mr. Goodbody," *Rolling Stone*, June 9, 1983.

188–89 **"To be even a passable model":** Sabol, *Body of America*, 72.

189   **1983 *New York Times* feature:** Judy Klemesrud, "Gym Clothes: Exercises in Style," *New York Times*, March 2, 1983, https://www.nytimes.com/1983/03/02/garden/gym-clothes-exercises-in-style.html.

189   **Roberts's family was Jewish:** Roberts's biographical section based primarily on the *New York Times* coverage of her life at the time of her death: Douglas Martin, "Lucille Roberts, 59, Founder of Fitness Chain for Women," *New York Times*, July 18, 2003, https://www.nytimes.com/2003/07/18/nyregion/lucille-roberts-59-founder-of-fitness-chain-for-women.html; Susan Dominus, "Ladies of the Gym Unite!" *New York Times*, December 28, 2003, https://www.nytimes.com/2003/12/28/magazine/the-lives-they-lived-ladies-of-the-gym-unite.html.

190   **"It is only the upper classes":** Edward Lewine, "The Fitness Gurus," *New York Times*, November 30, 1997, https://www.nytimes.com/1997/11/30/nyregion/the-fitness-gurus.html.

190   **"[taking] their cues from country clubs":** Shelly McKenzie, *Getting Physical: The Rise of Fitness Culture in America* (University Press of Kansas, 2013), 174.

191   **Gyms continued to discriminate:** McKenzie, *Getting Physical*, 174–75.

191 **As *Sports Illustrated* noted in 1984:** Jack McCallum, "Everybody's Doin' It," *Sports Illustrated*, December 3, 1984, https://vault.si.com/vault/1984/12/03/everybodys-doin-it.

191 **In 1982, the beloved Jane Fonda Workout instructor:** Janice Darling, interview with the author, April 20, 2021.

192 **The story behind "Physical":** See Olivia Newton-John, *Olivia Newton-John: Don't Stop Believin'* (Gallery Books, 2018), 177–83, Apple Books; Madison Vain, "What Made Olivia Newton-John 'Horrified' About 'Physical,'" *Entertainment Weekly*, April 13, 2017, https://ew.com/music/2017/04/13/olivia-newton-john-physical-interview/.

194 **"To be in condition":** Corliss, "Coming on Strong."

194 **"superficial appearances really can be equated":** Susan J. Douglas, *Where the Girls Are: Growing Up Female with the Mass Media* (Three Rivers Press, 1994), 260.

194 **"Now all the world was a gym":** Sabol, *Body of America,* 64.

195 **"Linda, you are ripped to shreds":** Jeanne Wolf, "Working Out with the Stars," *Cosmopolitan*, May 1992, 243.

195 **women wanted them:** See, for example, "The Ultimate Upper-Body Workout," *Ladies' Home Journal*, April 1992, 38, 42, featuring Linda Hamilton's trainer.

195 **"a signal to one another":** Kara Jesella, "The Collarbone's Connected to Slimness," *New York Times*, May 10, 2007, https://www.nytimes.com/2007/05/10/fashion/10clavicle.html.

196 **Tamilee Webb grew up:** Tamilee Webb biographical sections drawn from Webb's interview with the author, October 21, 2020.

198 ***Buns of Steel* brand initially began:** *Buns of Steel* origin story and the quotes therein drawn from the author's interview with Webb, October 21, 2020, and with Melissa McNeese, former head of marketing for the Maier Group, April 22, 2020.

200 **By 1993, Tamilee's videos:** "Top Special Interest Video Sales, Health & Fitness," *Billboard*, June 12, 1993, 63; see also Peter M. Nichols, "Home Video," *New York Times*, September 3, 1993, https://www.nytimes.com/1993/09/03/arts/home-video-952393.html.

200 **10 million copies:** Webb, interview, October 21, 2020.

200 **a volume of *Cathy* cartoons:** Cathy Guisewite, *Abs of Steel, Buns of Cinnamon* (Andrews McMeel Publishing, 1997).

202 **"better thighs":** Douglas, *Where the Girls Are*, 263.

202 **"oozes menacingly"**: Randall Rothenberg, "A Lighthearted Look At Being Overweight," *New York Times*, September 6, 1989, https://www.nytimes.com/1989/09/06/business/the-media-business-advertising-a-lighthearted-look-at-being-overweight.html.

202 **Somers told *Entrepreneur*:** Dan Bova, "Suzanne Somers Explains How ThighMaster Squeezed Its Way Into Infomercial History," *Entrepreneur*, June 25, 2020, https://www.entrepreneur.com/article/352389.

202 **"the ultimate signifier":** Douglas, *Where the Girls Are*, 258.

203 **"reintroduce weakness":** Steinem, *Moving Beyond Words*, 97.

204 **my fitness bible:** Jessica Vitkus, *Beauty and Fitness with Saved by the Bell* (Aladdin, 1992), page 17.

204 **Tracy James:** See https://www.tracyjames.com/biography.html.

205 **But then two months go by:** J. C. Herz, *Learning to Breathe Fire: The Rise of CrossFit and the Primal Future of Fitness* (Crown Archetype, 2014), 68, Kindle.

205 **Shannon Wagner, founder of the Women's Strength Coalition:** Shannon Wagner, interview with the author for Medium's Forge, September 18, 2019. See https://forge.medium.com/what-happens-when-women-start-taking-up-space-4ce5a3206853.

206 **"For hundreds of years":** Shapley, *Strong Like Her*, 180.

Chapter 7 | Stretch

207 **"Wanna fly":** Toni Morrison, *Song of Solomon* (Vintage, 1977), 179, Kindle.

208 **"Basically, we all need":** Blair Sabol, *The Body of America: An Insider's Journey Through the Bumps & Pumps, Groans & Moans, Pecs & Wrecks, Sweat & Sex of the Fitness Explosion* (Arbor House, 1986), 223.

208 **was decreasing:** Shelly McKenzie, *Getting Physical: The Rise of Fitness Culture in America* (University Press of Kansas, 2013), 176.

208 **"After years of bowing":** Alicia Lasek, "Kathy Smith Is Adding Yoga to Her Videocassette Library. Superwoman's Dead Fitness Craze Goes Softer; Walking and Gardening Blossom," *AdAge*, November 7, 1994, https://adage.com/article/news/kathy-smith-adding-yoga-videocassette-library-superwoman-s-dead-fitness-craze-softer-walking-gardening-blossom/89398.

209 **number of Americans:** Julie Jacob, "Think About Your Next Move," *Chicago Tribune*, August 4, 2002, https://www.chicagotribune.com/news/ct-xpm-2002-08-04-0208040337-story.html.

209   **"gone mainstream":** *U.S. News & World Report* cover line, May 16, 1994.

209   **Indra Devi:** Essential sources for Devi biographical sections include Indra Devi, *Forever Young, Forever Healthy* (Prentice-Hall, 1953); Michelle Goldberg, *The Goddess Pose: The Audacious Life of Indra Devi, the Woman Who Helped Bring Yoga to the West* (Alfred A. Knopf, 2015), Kindle; Stefanie Syman, *The Subtle Body: The Story of Yoga in America* (Farrar, Straus and Giroux, 2010), 187, Kindle; Janice Gates, *Yogini: The Power of Women in Yoga* (Mandala Publishing, 2006), 45–48; Audrey Youngman, "The Grande Dame of Yoga," *Yoga Journal*, September/October 1996, 74–79, 146–48, https://books.google.com/books?id=WekDAAAAMBAJ&pg=PA2&source=gbs_toc&cad=2#v=onepage&q=indra%20devi&f=false; and Douglas Martin, "Indra Devi, 102, Dies; Taught Yoga to Stars and Leaders," *New York Times*, April 30, 2002, https://www.nytimes.com/2002/04/30/world/indra-devi-102-dies-taught-yoga-to-stars-and-leaders.html.

210   **"esoteric female Forrest":** Goldberg, *The Goddess Pose*, 8.

210   **"As a child, I intuited":** As cited in Goldberg, *The Goddess Pose*, 13.

210   **"plagued by inexplicable terrors":** Goldberg, *The Goddess Pose*, 16.

211   **She listened "breathlessly":** Devi, *Forever Young, Forever Healthy*, 3.

211   **It was only later:** Goldberg, *The Goddess Pose*, 19.

211   **"India was to me the land":** Devi, *Forever Young, Forever Healthy*, 6.

211   **"She was only one letter away":** Goldberg, *The Goddess Pose*, 83.

211   **"Comfortably married":** Devi, *Forever Young, Forever Healthy*, 9.

212   **"I wasn't actually *doing* anything else":** Devi, *Forever Young, Forever Healthy*, 9.

212   **"When educated people":** Goldberg, *The Goddess Pose*, 96.

212   **"This old and typical":** Goldberg, *The Goddess Pose*, 90.

213   **"devoted to spreading":** Goldberg, *The Goddess Pose*, 120.

213   **"He was very strict with me":** Youngman, "The Grande Dame of Yoga," 76.

213   **"numerous disparate sources":** Syman, *The Subtle Body*, 187.

213   **"Inside of a few months":** Devi, *Forever Young, Forever Healthy*, 19.

214   **"When my teacher saw":** Devi, *Forever Young, Forever Healthy*, 19.

215   **"I decided to leave the matter":** Youngman, "The Grande Dame of Yoga," 79.

215   **Violent crime was at an all-time high:** Syman, *The Subtle Body*, 179.

215 **"a great hunger":** Goldberg, *The Goddess Pose*, 157.

215 **lavish private villa:** Goldberg, *The Goddess Pose*, 156–57.

216 **"She had no job":** Goldberg, *The Goddess Pose*, 157.

216 **"The only thing left to do":** As cited in Goldberg, *The Goddess Pose*, 157.

216 **Outside, she planted a wood sign:** Syman, *The Subtle Body*, 180; for a visual, see https://www.gettyimages.com/detail/news-photo/student-walks-to-indra-devi-yoga-studio-in-hollywood-news-photo/596709037?adppopup=true.

216 **1951 advertisement for Jergens:** Syman, *The Subtle Body*, 189; see advertisement: Jergens, *Good Housekeeping*, February 1951, 5.

217 **"[She] went to great pains":** Goldberg, *The Goddess Pose*, 163.

217 **flowing shorts:** See Devi, *Forever Young, Forever Healthy*, 16.

217 **"Devi was both gracious and exacting":** Syman, *The Subtle Body*, 180.

217 **"How often do you take yogurt?":** Devi, *Forever Young, Forever Healthy*, 23.

218 **"She wanted me to join her staff":** Youngman, "The Grande Dame of Yoga," 79.

218 **"Under the 'veil' of yoga,":** Goldberg, *The Goddess Pose*, 164–65.

218 **"Devi was a Russian with multiple aliases":** Goldberg, *The Goddess Pose*, 165.

219 **"This book is written":** Devi, *Forever Young*, ix.

219 **strikingly candid about sex:** Devi, *Forever Young*, 107–16.

219 **"grants woman equality":** Devi, *Forever Young*, 119.

219 **"The Woman Beautiful":** Devi, *Forever Young*, 117–18.

220 **"keep the body healthy, beautiful":** Devi, *Forever Young*, 27.

221 **"teach him some deep-breathing exercises":** Goldberg, *The Goddess Pose*, 194.

221 **"She doesn't seem to have had a plan":** Goldberg, *The Goddess Pose*, 197.

222 **Counterculture icons:** See Syman, *The Subtle Body*, "Chapter 10: Psychedelic Sages," 198–232; Natalia Mehlman Petrzela, PhD, "The Siren Song of Yoga: Sex, Spirituality, and the Limits of American Countercultures," *Pacific Historical Review* 89, no. 3 (summer 2020): 379–401, https://online.ucpress.edu/phr/article-abstract/89/3/379/110887/The-Siren-Song-of-Yoga-Sex-Spirituality-and-the?redirectedFrom=fulltext.

222 **"Everybody's talking about yoga":** Beverly Wilson, "Yoga for All: The First Lesson," *Los Angeles Times*, January 8, 1961.

222 **"I was first introduced":** Joe Hyams, Herald Tribune News Service, "Hittleman's Taking Yoga to the Ladies," *Washington Post*, August 2, 1961.

223 **"ancient beauty secret":** "Yoga: Ancient Beauty Secret," *Seventeen*, November 1961, 100–101.

223 ***Cosmopolitan* ran a feature:** Jess Stern, "How Yoga Can Change Your Life," *Cosmopolitan*, September 1965, 44–51.

223 ***Seventeen* pitched it:** "Yoga: Ancient Beauty Secret," *Seventeen*.

224 **"yoga was something the hippies":** Syman, *The Subtle Body*, 234.

224 **"Yoga is not just for Eastern mystics":** Boston Women's Health Book Collective, *Our Bodies, Ourselves: A Book By and For Women* (Simon & Schuster, 1971), 117.

224 **the "Julia Child of Yoga":** "Modern Living: Beating the Blahs," *Time*, October 7, 1974, http://content.time.com/time/subscriber/article/0,33009,943051,00 .html.

224 **Three times a week, Lilias Folan:** Lilias Folan biographical section draws primarily from the author's interview with Folan on February 11, 2021; "Modern Living: Beating the Blahs," *Time*; and Gates, *Yogini*, 61–66.

225 **at the top of a 1974 episode:** "Lilias, Yoga and You," Public Broadcasting Service, 1974. Shared on Vimeo by Folan's son, Michael Folan, https:// vimeo.com/channels/443007/59686744.

226 **"If you want a beautiful or handsome body":** Lilas Folan, *Lilias, Yoga and You* (WCET-TV, 1972), 5.

226 **"I've fallen head over heels":** Gerald Nachman, "A Love That's Shaping Up," *San Francisco Chronicle*, August 29, 1979, https://www.sfgate.com /entertainment/article/A-love-that-s-shaping-up-4184647.php.

227 **one woman commented:** "Lilias Yoga and You—'The Fish Pose,'" Vimeo, viewer comment, https://vimeo.com/channels/443007/59686744.

227 **"This was the missing media link":** Syman, *The Subtle Body*, 245.

227 **rise of modern yoga mats:** See Fernando Pages Ruiz, "The Sticky Business + History of Yoga Mats," *Yoga Journal*, August 28, 2007, https://www .yogajournal.com/yoga-101/sticky-business/.

228 **"Aerobics emphasized power and strength":** Syman, *The Subtle Body*, 265.

228 **In 1984, *Sports Illustrated* sat in:** Jack McCallum, "Everybody's Doin' It," *Sports Illustrated*, December 3, 1984, https://vault.si.com/vault/1984 /12/03/everybodys-doin-it.

228 **called the "Harvey Weinstein of Yoga":** See, for example: Carly Mallenbaum, "Why Bikram Yoga's Founder Is in Hot Water in a New Netflix Documentary," *USA Today*, November 22, 2019, https://www.usatoday .com/story/entertainment/movies/2019/11/22/bikram-yoga-founder -under-fire-new-netflix-documentary-heres-why/4250553002/.

229 **Jivamukti yoga center:** See Penelope Green, "Modern Yoga: Om to the Beat," *New York Times*, March 15, 1998, https://www.nytimes.com/1998 /03/15/style/view-modern-yoga-om-to-the-beat.html, and Linda Solomon, "Living the High Life at Jivamukti," *Yoga Journal*, September/October 1998, 72–75, 136.

229 **Raquel Welch published:** Raquel Welch, *Raquel: The Raquel Welch Total Beauty and Fitness Program* (Ballantine, 1984).

229 **Allison Yarrow calls the "bitchification":** Allison Yarrow, *90s Bitch: Media, Culture, and the Failed Promise of Gender Equality* (Harper Perennial, 2018), viii, Kindle.

230 **"It's the '90s and the woman appears":** Solomon, "Living the High Life."

230 **"The yoga body—":** Green, "Modern Yoga."

230 **Oprah demonstrated asanas:** Anne Cushman, "If Yoga's Chic, Does that Mean I Am, Too?" *Yoga Journal*, September/October 1998, 76–79.

230 **"Yoga now straddles the continent":** Richard Corliss, "The Power of Yoga," *Time*, April 15, 2001, http://content.time.com/time/health/article /0,8599,106356,00.html.

230 **"Like any other force":** Cushman, "If Yoga's Chic."

231 ***Yoga Journal* co-founder Judith Lasater:** Gates, *Yogini*, 90.

232 **more than $37 billion:** "Yoga Market by Type (Online Yoga Course, Offline Yoga Course, and Yoga Accreditation Training Programs): Global Opportunity Analysis and Industry Forecast, 2021–2027," Allied Market Research, October 7, 2020, https://www.prnewswire.com/news-releases/yoga -market-to-reach-66-22-bn-globally-by-2027-at-9-6-cagr-amr-301147486 .html.

232 **"Those without access":** Rina Deshpande, "What's the Difference Between Cultural Appropriation and Cultural Appreciation?" *Yoga Journal*, May 1, 2019, https://www.yogajournal.com/yoga-101/yoga-cultural-appropriation -appreciation/.

234   **36 million Americans:** See "2016 Yoga in America Study Conducted by Yoga Journal and Yoga Alliance," https://www.yogaalliance.org/2016 YogaInAmericaStudy.

234   **When I spoke with Judith Lasater:** Judith Lasater (co-founding editor of *Yoga Journal*), interview with the author, February 23, 2021.

Chapter 8 | Expand

235   **"We are not meant to be perfect":** See "Jane Fonda on Perfection," Oprah's Master Class, Opera Winfrey Network, January 9, 2012, https://www.youtube.com/watch?v=A4AnHAwHQB4.

235   **"To be rather than to seem":** See Michael Parker, "To Be Rather Than to Seem: North Carolina's State Motto," Our State, July 2, 2014, https://www.ourstate.com/state-motto/.

237   **Regular exercise improves:** For a summary of the benefits, see https://www.who.int/news-room/fact-sheets/detail/physical-activity.

237   **"Movement is intertwined":** Kelly McGonigal, *The Joy of Movement: How Exercise Helps Us Find Happiness, Hope, Connection, and Courage* (Avery, 2019), 6–7.

237   **Only a quarter of Americans:** Tainya C. Clarke, Tina Norris, and Jeannine S. Schiller, "Early Release of Selected Estimates Based on Data from the National Health Interview Survey," National Center for Health Statistics, May 2019; available from https://www.cdc.gov/nchs/nhis.htm.

237   **In 2019, Americans paid:** International Health, Racquet & Sportsclub Association, 2018 IHRSA Health Club Media Report, released December 2017, 18.

237   **"The opportunity to engage in physical activity":** Ophelia Yeung and Katherine Johnston, Global Wellness Institute, "Move to Be Well: The Global Economy of Physical Activity," October 2019, 17, https://globalwellnessinstitute.org/wp-content/uploads/2020/09/GWI_2019_Global-Economy-of-Physical-Activity_North-America_Download.pdf.

238   **"The formalization of exercise":** Shelly McKenzie, *Getting Physical: The Rise of Fitness Culture in America* (University Press of Kansas, 2013), 179.

238   **"To most people":** McKenzie, *Getting Physical*, 181.

240   **"one-woman visibility crusader":** Lindsay Tucker, "Jessamyn Stanley on Moving Beyond Body Positivity," *Yoga Journal*, December 21, 2018, https://www.yogajournal.com/lifestyle/jessamyn-stanley-moving-beyond-body-positivity/.

240   **"Burning Down the House"**: See *Yoga Journal*, January 2019, 78, https://www.yogajournallibrary.com/view/issue/307/page/79/#page=78.

240   **"authorship of how we were seen"**: Virgie Tovar, interview with the author for Medium's Forge, October 8, 2019. See https://forge.medium.com/what-happens-when-women-start-taking-up-space-4ce5a3206853.

241   **Jessamyn wouldn't have risen:** Essential references for Stanley biographical sections include the author's interview with Stanley, March 10, 2021; Jessamyn Stanley, *Every Body Yoga: Let Go of Fear, Get On the Mat, Love Your Body* (Workman Publishing Co., 2017), Kindle; and Tucker, "Jessamyn Stanley."

241   **"I was practicing yoga at home"**: Stanley, interview, March 10, 2021.

241   **"wide nose, big belly"**: Lottie Lumsden and Annabelle Lee, "11 women who prove wellness isn't 'one size fits all,'" *Cosmopolitan UK*, January 1, 2021, https://www.cosmopolitan.com/uk/body/a34915032/women-bodies-wellness-healthy-different-shape-size/.

241   **"I'd sustained enough"**: Stanley, *Every Body Yoga*, 200.

242   **"Even though I knew my looks"**: Stanley, *Every Body Yoga*, 214.

242   **"epitome of glamour"**: Stanley, *Every Body Yoga*, 16.

242   **"In a room full of"**: Stanley, *Every Body Yoga*, 16.

243   **"I couldn't deny"**: Stanley, *Every Body Yoga*, 18.

243   **"I remember feeling as though"**: Stanley, *Every Body Yoga*, 19.

243   **"That was a triumph all my own"**: Stanley, *Every Body Yoga*, 21.

244   **That's when everything changed:** Stanley, *Every Body Yoga*, 7.

244   **"I couldn't have anticipated"**: Stanley, *Every Body Yoga*, 255.

244   **"'I didn't know fat people could do yoga'"**: Tucker, "Jessamyn Stanley."

245   **"I wrote this book"**: Stanley, *Every Body Yoga*, 7.

245   **"I just practice trying to live my life"**: Stanley, interview, March 10, 2021.

246   **"Although I am frequently"**: Jenna Wortham, "Finding a More Inclusive Vision of Fitness in Our Feeds," *New York Times*, July 6, 2017, https://www.nytimes.com/2017/07/06/magazine/finding-a-more-inclusive-vision-of-fitness-in-our-feeds.html.

246   **During the pandemic:** Amira Rose Davis, interview with the author, April 14, 2021; see also L'Oreal Thompson Payton, "Inside the Peloton

Community Dedicated to Black Women," Zora, June 30, 2020, https://zora
.medium.com/inside-the-peloton-community-dedicated-to-black-women
-27f5c2a7064a.

246 **"I have never seen":** Davis, interview, April 14, 2021.

246 **research has shown:** Rodney P. Joseph et al., "Hair as a Barrier to Physical Activity Among African American Women: A Qualitative Exploration," *Frontiers in Public Health* 5 (January 17, 2018): 367; Linda Carroll,
"Hair Care Issues May Keep Some Black Women from Exercising," Re-
uters, November 11, 2019, https://www.reuters.com/article/us-health-fitness
-african-americans/hair-care-issues-may-keep-some-black-women
-from-exercising-idUSKBN1XL27R.

246 **uterine fibroids:** See Hilda Hutcherson, "Black Women Are Hit Hardest
by Fibroid Tumors," *New York Times*, April 15, 2020, https://www.nytimes
.com/2020/04/15/parenting/fertility/black-women-uterine-fibroids.html.

247 **radical body love:** See, for example: Maya Salam, "Why 'Radical Body
Love' Is Thriving on Instagram," *New York Times*, June 9, 2017, https://
www.nytimes.com/2017/06/09/style/body-positive-instagram.html.

247–48 **Research has shown time and again:** See Lindo Bacon, PhD, and Lucy
Aphramor, PhD, RD, *Body Respect: What Conventional Health Books Get
Wrong, Leave Out, and Just Plain Fail to Understand About Weight* (Ben-
Bella Books, 2014).

248 **Health at Every Size movement:** See https://haescommunity.com/; Bacon
and Aphramor, *Body Respect*.

248 **"reduces their ill health":** Bacon and Aphramor, *Body Respect*, location 242.

249 **"the gap between those weights":** Bacon and Aphramor, *Body Respect*, 17.

249 **"Across every category":** Bacon and Aphramor, *Body Respect*, location
16–17.

249 **"shift their focus away":** Bacon and Aphramor, *Body Respect*, 28.

249 **"When you tell a woman":** Tovar, interview, October 8, 2019.

250 **Cardio dance pioneer Sadie Kurzban:** Kurzban (founder of 305 Fitness), interview with the author, November 20, 2020.

251 **"I started 305 as a way":** Megan Bruneau, "From Disordered Eating to
Sexism, 305 Fitness Founder Sadie Kurzban Dances Through Challenge,"
Forbes, January 5, 2019, https://www.forbes.com/sites/meganbruneau/2019
/01/05/from-disordered-eating-to-sexism-how-305-fitness-founder-sadie
-kurzban-dances-through-challenge/.

252 **"The face of 305":** See Bruneau, "From Disordered Eating."

253 **The co-founders of Physique 57:** Jennifer Maanavi interview with the author, May 24, 2019; Tanya Becker interview with the author, June 16, 2019.

254 **"There's been a buy-in":** Elizabeth Matelski, PhD (associate professor of history at Endicott College; author, *Reducing Bodies*), interview with the author for Medium's Forge, September 16, 2019.

254 **"Either tactic, either motivation":** Tovar, interview, October 8, 2019.

255 **Elaine LaLanne:** Elaine LaLanne, interview with the author, November 25, 2019.

255 **Joyce Hein:** Joyce Hein, interview with the author, February 24, 2020.

256 **"Maybe in our Western culture":** Jane Fonda, *My Life So Far* (Random House, 2005), 745.

257 **"My mom had cheerleading":** Lindsay Crouse, "Inspiring Her Daughter, an Olympic Runner, Was No Sweat for a Fitness Guru," *New York Times*, August 17, 2016, https://www.nytimes.com/2016/08/17/sports/olympics/kate -grace-runner-kathy-smith-mother-inspiration.html.

258 **"Somehow the brain is tricked":** McGonigal, *Joy of Movement*, 74.

Where Are They Now?

259 **"Every once in a while":** Samantha Dunn, "Our Heroines," *Living Fit*, October 1997.

259 **took a final bow:** Bonnie's legacy lives on through the website bonnieprud den.com, which is overseen by Enid Whittaker.

259 **Lotte Berk continued:** Julie Welch, "Lotte Berk: Stylish Dancer Who Became a Fitness Icon," *Guardian*, November 8, 2003, https://www.theguardian .com/news/2003/nov/08/guardianobituaries.artsobituaries; Wolfgang Saxon, "Lotte Berk, 90, German Dancer Who Slimmed London's Stylish," *New York Times*, November 17, 2003, https://www.nytimes.com/2003/11/17 /world/lotte-berk-90-german-dancer-who-slimmed-london-s-stylish.html.

260 **The group uses running:** See https://www.261fearless.org/.

263 **The Bodyful Mind:** See https://thebodyfulmind.com/.

264 **legally adopted by Dr. John Lilly:** John Lombardi, "Little Miss Dangerous," *Spy*, October 1991.

Selected Bibliography

Bach, Lydia. *Awake! Aware! Alive! Exercises for a Vital Body.* New York: Random House, 1973.

Bacon, Lindo, PhD. *Health at Every Size: The Surprising Truth About Your Weight.* Dallas: BenBella Books, 2010.

Bacon, Lindo, PhD, and Lucy Aphramor, PhD, RD. *Body Respect: What Conventional Health Books Get Wrong, Leave Out, and Just Plain Fail to Understand About Weight.* Dallas: BenBella Books, 2014.

Black, Jonathan. *Making the American Body: The Remarkable Saga of the Men and Women Whose Feats, Feuds, and Passions Shaped Fitness History.* Lincoln: University of Nebraska Press, 2013.

Boston Women's Health Book Collective. *Our Bodies, Ourselves: A Book By and For Women.* New York: Simon & Schuster, 1971.

Bosworth, Patricia. *Jane Fonda: The Private Life of a Public Woman.* Boston: Houghton Mifflin Harcourt, 2011.

Brunberg, Joan Jacobs. *The Body Project: An Intimate History of American Girls*. New York: Random House, 1997.

Burfoot, Amby. *First Ladies of Running: 22 Inspiring Profiles of the Rebels, Rule Breakers, and Visionaries Who Changed the Sport Forever*. New York: Rodale Books, 2016.

Coontz, Stephanie. *A Strange Stirring: The* Feminine Mystique *and American Women at the Dawn of the 1960s*. New York: Basic Books, 2011.

Cooper, Kenneth H., MD. *Aerobics*. New York: M. Evans and Co., 1968.

Cooper, Mildred, and Kenneth H. Cooper, MD. *Aerobics for Women*. New York: M. Evans and Co., 1972.

Devi, Indra. *Forever Young, Forever Healthy*. Hoboken, NJ: Prentice Hall, 1953.

Douglas, Susan J. *Where the Girls Are: Growing Up Female with the Mass Media*. New York: Three Rivers Press, 1994.

Drake, Debbie. *Debbie Drake's Easy Way to a Perfect Figure and Glowing Health*. Hoboken, NJ: Prentice Hall, 1962.

Fairfax, Esther. *My Improper Mother and Me*. London: Central Books, 2010.

Folan, Lilias. *Lilias, Yoga and You*. Cincinnati, OH: WCET-TV, 1972.

Fonda, Jane. *Jane Fonda's Workout Book.* New York: Simon & Schuster, 1981.

———. *My Life So Far.* New York: Random House, 2005.

Gaines, Charles, and George Butler. *Pumping Iron II: The Unprecedented Woman.* New York: Simon & Schuster, 1984.

Gates, Janice. *Yogini: The Power of Women in Yoga.* New York: Mandala Publishing, 2006.

Gibb, Bobbi. *Wind in the Fire: The Personal Journey of the First Woman to Run the Boston Marathon.* Cambridge, MA: The Institute for the Study of Natural Systems Press, 2016.

Goldberg, Michelle. *The Goddess Pose: The Audacious Life of Indra Devi, the Woman Who Helped Bring Yoga to the West.* New York: Alfred A. Knopf, 2015.

Hauser, Brooke. *Enter Helen: The Invention of Helen Gurley Brown and the Rise of the Modern Single Woman.* New York: HarperCollins, 2016.

Jeffords, Susan. *Hard Bodies: Hollywood Masculinity in the Reagan Era.* New Brunswick, NJ: Rutgers University Press, 1993.

Kolata, Gina. *Ultimate Fitness: The Quest for Truth About Health and Exercise.* New York: Farrar, Straus and Giroux, 2003.

Kunitz, Daniel. *Lift: Fitness Culture, from Naked Greeks and Acrobats to Jazzercise and Ninja Warriors.* New York, Harper Wave, 2016.

Lindahl, Lisa. *Unleash the Girls: The Untold Story of the Invention of the Sports Bra and How It Changed the World (And Me)*. Charleston, SC: EZL Enterprises, 2019.

Lister, Jenny. *Mary Quant*. London: Victoria & Albert Museum; illustrated edition, 2019.

Lutter, Judy Mahle, and Lynn Jaffee. *The Bodywise Woman*. Champaign, IL: Human Kinetics, 1996.

Lyon, Lisa, and Douglas Kent Hall. *Lisa Lyon's Body Magic: A Total Program of Body Conditioning by the First World Women's Bodybuilding Champion*. New York: Bantam, 1981.

MacCambridge, Michael. *The Franchise: A History of* Sports Illustrated *Magazine*. New York: Hyperion, 1997.

Mapplethorpe, Robert; text by Bruce Chatwin. *Lady: Lisa Lyon*. New York: Viking, 1983.

Marx, Gilda. *Body by Gilda: Redesign Every Line*. New York: G. P. Putnam's Sons, 1984.

Matelski, Elizabeth. *Reducing Bodies: Mass Culture and the Female Figure in Postwar America*. New York: Routledge, 2017.

McGonigal, Kelly, PhD. *The Joy of Movement: How Exercise Helps Us Find Happiness, Hope, Connection, and Courage*. New York: Avery, 2019.

McKenzie, Shelly. *Getting Physical: The Rise of Fitness Culture in America*. Lawrence: University Press of Kansas, 2013.

Meltzer, Marisa. *This Is Big: How the Founder of Weight Watchers Changed the World—and Me*. New York: Little, Brown, 2020.

Missett, Judi Sheppard. *Building a Business with a Beat: Leadership Lessons from Jazzercise—An Empire Built on Passion, Purpose, and Heart*. New York: McGraw-Hill, 2019.

Missett, Judi Sheppard, with Donna Z. Meilach. *Jazzercise: A Fun Way to Fitness: America's Popular New Way to Fitness . . . Easy Dance-Exercises Set to the Rhythms of Jazz*. New York: Bantam Books, 1978.

O'Connor, Kaori. *Lycra: How a Fiber Shaped America*. New York: Routledge, 2011.

Prudden, Bonnie. *How to Keep Slender and Fit After Thirty*. New York: Bernard Geis Associates, 1961.

Quant, Mary. *Quant by Quant*. New York: G. P. Putnam's Sons, 1966.

Sabol, Blair. *The Body of America: An Insider's Journey Through the Bumps & Pumps, Groans & Moans, Pecs & Wrecks, Sweat & Sex of the Fitness Explosion*. New York: Arbor House, 1986.

Schulman, Bruce J. *The Seventies: The Great Shift in American Culture, Society, and Politics*. New York: The Free Press, 2001.

Schultz, Jaime. *Qualifying Times: Points of Change in U.S. Women's Sports*. Champaign: University of Illinois Press, 2014.

Shapley, Haley. *Strong Like Her: A Celebration of Rule Breakers, History Makers, and Unstoppable Athletes*. New York: Gallery Books, 2020.

Smith, Nicholas. *Kicks: The Great American Story of Sneakers*. New York: Crown, 2018.

Stanley, Jessamyn. *Every Body Yoga: Let Go of Fear, Get On the Mat, Love Your Body*. New York: Workman Publishing, 2017.

Steinem, Gloria. *Moving Beyond Words: Essays on Age, Rage, Sex, Power, Money, Muscles: Breaking the Boundaries of Gender*. New York: Simon & Schuster, 1994.

———. *Revolution from Within: A Book of Self-Esteem*. New York: Little, Brown, 1992.

Strings, Sabrina. *Fearing the Black Body: The Racial Origins of Fat Phobia*. New York: New York University Press, 2019.

Swaby, Rachel, and Kit Fox. *Mighty Moe: The True Story of a Thirteen-Year-Old Running Revolutionary*. New York: Farrar, Straus Giroux Books for Young Readers, 2019.

Swanson, Beth S. "A History of the Rise of Aerobic Dance in the United States Through 1980." Master's thesis, San Jose State University, 1996.

Switzer, Kathrine. *Marathon Woman: Running the Race to Revolutionize Women's Sports.* New York: Da Capo Press, 2009.

Syman, Stefanie. *The Subtle Body: The Story of Yoga in America.* New York: Farrar, Straus and Giroux, 2010.

Warner, Judith. *Perfect Madness: Motherhood in the Age of Anxiety.* New York: Riverhead, 2005.

Photo Credits

Prudden demonstrates trampoline exercises: Orlando/Three Lions/ Getty Images.

Prudden gets down to business: Susan Wood/Getty Images.

Lotte Berk, creator of the barre workout: Courtesy of Esther Fairfax.

Berk lounges in the garden: Courtesy of Esther Fairfax.

Berk with her daughter: Courtesy of Esther Fairfax.

Berk shows off her first sports car: Courtesy of Esther Fairfax.

Boston Marathon co-director Jock Semple: *Boston Herald*/Courtesy of Kathrine Switzer and 261 Fearless.

Bobbi Gibb barrels toward the finish line: Fred Kaplan/*Sports Illustrated*/ Getty Images.

Switzer at the start of New York: *Marathon Woman: Running the Race to Revolutionize Women's Sports* by Kathrine Switzer.

Advertisement for the first modern sports bra: Jogbra, Inc. records, Archives Center, National Museum of American History, Smithsonian Institution.

Jazzercise creator Judi Sheppard Missett: Courtesy of Jazzercise Inc.

Missett leads a Jazzercise class: Courtesy of Jazzercise Inc.

Flexatard designer Gilda Marx: Courtesy of Gilda Marx.

Leni Cazden, the original architect: Courtesy of Tama Rothschild and Leni Cazden.

Jane Fonda at the opening: Ron Galella/Ron Galella Collection/Getty Images.

Janice Darling taught at the original: Courtesy of Steve Smith (stevesmithphotography.com) and Janice Darling.

Fonda feels the burn: Steve Schapiro/Corbis/Getty Images.

Bodybuilding pioneer Lisa Lyon: Douglas Kent Hall/Courtesy of Dawn Hall/Special Collections, Princeton University Library.

When she was crowned Ms. Olympia: Ron Galella/Ron Galella Collection/Getty Images.

A student visits the Indra Devi: Earl Leaf/Michael Ochs Archives/Getty Images.

Devi instructs the student: Earl Leaf/Michael Ochs Archives/Getty Images.

Yoga teacher Lilias Folan: Duane Howell/*The Denver Post*/Getty Images.

Folan lets loose with Phil Donahue: Courtesy of Lilias Folan.

Yoga teacher and Instagram star Jessamyn Stanley: Bobby Quillard/Courtesy of Jessamyn Stanley.

305 Fitness founder Sadie Kurzban: Courtesy of 305 Fitness.

Kurzban instructs a 305 Fitness class: Courtesy of 305 Fitness.

Index

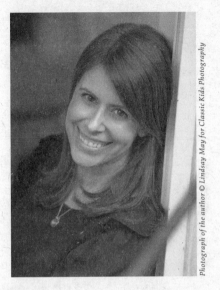

Photograph of the author © Lindsay May for Classic Kids Photography

Danielle Friedman is an award-winning journalist whose writing has appeared in *The New York Times, The Cut, Vogue, Harper's Bazaar, Glamour, Health, Time,* and other publications. She has worked as a senior editor at NBC News Digital and *The Daily Beast,* and she began her career as a nonfiction book editor at the Penguin imprints Hudson Street Press and Plume. She lives in New York City with her husband and son.

VISIT DANIELLE FRIEDMAN ONLINE

Danielle-Friedman.com
🐦 @DFriedmanWrites
📷 @DanielleFriedmanWrites